Neurocultural Health and Wellbeing

Series Editors
Lorenzo Lorusso, Neurology Unit, A.S.S.T. Lecco-Merate, Merate, Italy
Bruno Colombo, DIMER, Neurologia, Ospedale San Raffaele, Milano, Italy
Alessandro Porro, Dip. di Scienze Cliniche e di Comunità, University of Milan, Milano, Italy
Nicholas Wade, Department of Psychology, University of Dundee, Dundee, UK

Aim of this devoted book Series in neurology is to highlight the relationship between neuroscience and culture. Nowadays, there is more evidence of how our brain is influenced by the various artistic and cultural disciplines, both in the form of entertainment as well as – and above all – through the emotions and gratification which lead to wellbeing. The emotional mechanisms, the different cultural manifestations provided, are due to the activation of a perceptual and cognitive range that constitute the basis of the social behaviors. All this makes us aware of the benefits the arts have on personal and collective health.

This concept was already known to philosophers in ancient times, who were convinced that inner balance was influenced by culture and in particular by music.

During the centuries, men understood that the *cultivation of the spirit*, or *humanitas*, had a certain role on behavior and from the beginning of modern experimental science, in the fifteenth, the spread of the notions of neuroanatomy allowed artists to get closer to the knowledge of the brain's mechanisms and reveal the emotional and empathic responses at the basis of creativity, and indeed of their own psychophysical wellbeing. A dialogue between the science of the mind and artistic disciplines was born. The results of this meeting made it possible to better define which mental processes are involved when we come into contact with the various humanistic disciplines, and how they can be applied, for instance, to the treatment of mental disorders and neuropsychiatric diseases.

The goal of this Series is both to prove the role of biological brain mechanisms and the influence of various artistic forms on clinical practice, especially in neuro-psychiatric disorders, as well as to trace different therapeutic and psycho-physical well-being applications based on scientific evidence from medical literature.

Volumes of the Series will be edited by experts under the supervision of an international editorial committee. Each book, focused on a specific discipline, will provide knowledge on relationship between the brain activity and different forms of language, communication, art. This close inter-relationship with specific focus on different forms of art will explain the effectiveness of this kind of approaches in neuro-psychiatric diseases.

This Series will allow to understand how the culture is one of the fundamental tools to improve general well-being, quality of life and motivation in neurological diseases.

This Series also find a correlation with SDG3 goal "ensuring healthy lives and promoting wellbeing for all at all ages" for the progress of the health and wellbeing considering that neurological diseases are on the rise worldwide including in the developing countries.

Francesco Brigo

Charcot's Lesson

Learning Scientific Reasoning and Clinical Methodology

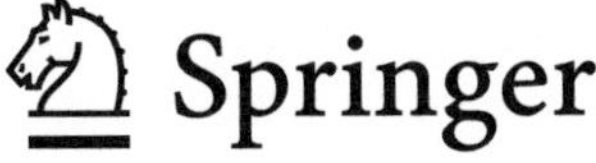 Springer

Francesco Brigo
Innovation, Research and Teaching Service (SABES-ASDAA)
Teaching Hospital of the Paracelsus Medical Private University (PMU)
Bolzano, Italy

ISSN 2731-4464   ISSN 2731-4472   (electronic)
Neurocultural Health and Wellbeing
ISBN 978-3-031-71223-4   ISBN 978-3-031-71221-0   (eBook)
https://doi.org/10.1007/978-3-031-71221-0

This Springer imprint is published by the registered company Springer Nature Switzerland AG
The registered company address is: Gewerbestrasse 11, 6330 Cham, Switzerland

If disposing of this product, please recycle the paper.

Preface

Ever since I can remember, I have been profoundly curious and fascinated by history. My father recalls that when I was between 4 and 5 years old, I was captivated by stories of Pharaohs, ancient Egypt, and Greek mythology, confidently engaging in conversations with adults on these topics. You can imagine how exasperating I must have been! As I grew older, my insatiable curiosity led me to explore other areas of human knowledge. Initially, I intended to pursue ancient Latin and Greek or philosophy at university. Given my complete lack of practical sense, if I had followed that path, I would likely be completely broke today. Instead, I eventually chose to study medicine and become a neurologist. Being a know-it-all and boringly meticulous, it is no surprise that I ended up in a field of medicine characterized by a very rigorous and precise method. To complicate matters, I developed an increasing interest in evidence-based practice and clinical methodology, deriving a certain pleasure from critically appraising scientific papers and scrutinizing everyone around me, whether peers, superiors, or even family members. In short, I became someone to avoid, always ready to identify flaws and inaccuracies.

As a result, my social appeal suffered considerably, but over time, I learned to critically evaluate my own thoughts and actions. Unexpectedly, I became more patient with those around me, acknowledging my own shortcomings before addressing those of others. My growing interest in methodology deepened my self-awareness and logical thinking, providing me with a framework to minimize errors or become more conscious of them. After all, the term "method" is derived from the ancient Greek word *metà—odòn*, meaning "along the way." Delving more and more in clinical methodology allowed me to follow the straight path. Not necessarily the shortest or most linear path, but one that proved the most effective in preventing as much as possible bad encounters and ruinous falls.

Along this path, I encountered many people who have been my steadfast companions and guiding lights. They supported me through the challenges and helped me steer clear of mental shortcuts and logical pitfalls. Among them, Ettore Beghi, a brilliant neuroepidemiologist, profoundly shaped my perspective on science and medicine. He imparted to me the importance of methodology, curiosity, and dedication, always infused with deep humanity.

Yet, another encounter along the way reignited my longstanding passion for history, now intertwined with my recent fascination with methodology. His name was

Jean-Martin Charcot, though I never met him, as he had passed away almost a century before I was born.

Strangely enough, my introduction to Charcot prompted profound reflections on key aspects of clinical reasoning and methodology. Like many, Charcot was not infallible; he was imperfect yet curious, aware of science's limitations, and committed to the asymptotic pursuit of truth, which can be approached without ever being fully reached. Despite (or perhaps because of) this, he dedicated his life to developing, systematizing, and refining the clinical method that continues to underpin modern neurology and can be applied across medical disciplines.

Charcot was not merely an academic figure; the transcripts of his engaging lectures at the Salpêtrière Hospital in Paris, where he interacted with patients, provide a vivid insight into the health and diseases of his time and offer a window into his method of reasoning. Over the years, my acquaintance with Charcot deepened, and I came to consider him not only as the father of modern neurology but also as one of the pioneers in clinical methodology.

One day, seemingly out of nowhere, I conceived the idea of writing a book recounting the wonders and challenges I encountered while exploring the path of clinical methodology alongside Charcot, a man who lived in a past century, spoke a different language, and whom I knew only through his writings.

This book explores key aspects of clinical methodology, evidence-based practice, and cognitive biases, using Jean-Martin Charcot's lectures as a starting point for discussion and in-depth analysis. My goal was to build a bridge between the illustrious and enduring legacy of the past and the contributions made by recent advances in epistemology and clinical methodology, drawing upon examples from Charcot's lectures as vivid and authentic illustrations to initiate discussions on various topics of interest.

This book covers a wide array of topics, including inductive and deductive reasoning, logical fallacies, the significance of history-taking, the Bayesian approach to diagnosis, principles of evidence-based practice, critical appraisal of clinical data, and the importance of maintaining a skeptical stance towards tradition and authority. Special emphasis is placed on cognitive biases and errors that commonly affect everyday clinical reasoning, with suggested strategies for recognizing and mitigating them to improve clinical activities and methodology.

Structured into concise chapters, each addressing a specific aspect, the book was neither conceived nor written in a linear manner, allowing it to be read cover-to-cover or in sections at the reader's discretion.

Throughout my exploration of clinical reasoning and methodology, I have sought to recount the challenging journey and convey the vastness of the panorama one could get from the mountaintop. Charcot has been an engaging companion on this journey. It is my hope that this book will inspire in you the desire to embark on your own journey with curiosity and openness, recognizing that each path is not merely a means to an end, but an enriching experience in itself.

And thus, we do approach the study of these dreadful maladies with prudence, no doubt, but also with confidence. We are permeated with the surety of the observation methods we have at hand.

—Jean-Martin Charcot, Leçons sur les Maladies du Système Nerveux faites a la Salpêtrière. Volume 3, Lecture I. Paris, 1883

Bolzano, Italy   Francesco Brigo

Contents

Part III   Epilogue

Part I
Methodological Aspects

Charcot, the Master: Who Was He and What Can We Learn from Him?

1

Jean-Martin Charcot (1825–1893) was a prominent French physician, widely revered as the father of modern neurology (Fig. 1.1). His lectures at the Salpêtrière Hospital in Paris, where he observed and treated patients with various neurological disorders, were meticulously transcribed and remain invaluable sources of insight into his clinical reasoning, diagnostic acumen, and methodological innovations, which continue to resonate in contemporary medical practice.

Charcot was a pioneer in the field of clinical reasoning, profoundly influencing the evolution of neurology and psychology. Central to his approach was the anatomo-clinical method, which integrated clinical signs with postmortem anatomical findings. Initially, he meticulously documented clinical manifestations over time and, upon patients' death, conducted detailed autopsies of the brain and spinal cord. This approach enabled Charcot to establish robust clinical-anatomical correlations, defining structures responsible for both normal and pathological neurological signs. His methodological rigor laid the foundation for a novel classification of neurological diseases based on anatomical substrates.

Charcot's contributions to medicine and neurology are vast and enduring. He notably characterized amyotrophic lateral sclerosis, multiple sclerosis, and neurogenic arthropathy and distinguished between tremors associated with multiple sclerosis and Parkinson's disease. His seminal work on clinical reasoning and neurological disorders has left an indelible mark on medical science, reflected in numerous medical eponyms, including Charcot's disease, synonymous with amyotrophic lateral sclerosis.

The lectures of Charcot serve as a treasure trove of insights into his clinical reasoning and methodological innovations. They offer a unique historical perspective on the evolution of medicine and neurology, providing invaluable lessons for contemporary medical practitioners. Charcot's approach to clinical reasoning, characterized by a meticulous analysis of patient symptoms, systematic history taking, and

© The Author(s), under exclusive license to Springer Nature Switzerland AG 2024
F. Brigo, *Charcot's Lesson*, Neurocultural Health and Wellbeing,
https://doi.org/10.1007/978-3-031-71221-0_1

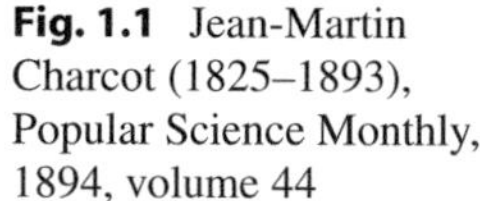

Fig. 1.1 Jean-Martin Charcot (1825–1893), Popular Science Monthly, 1894, volume 44

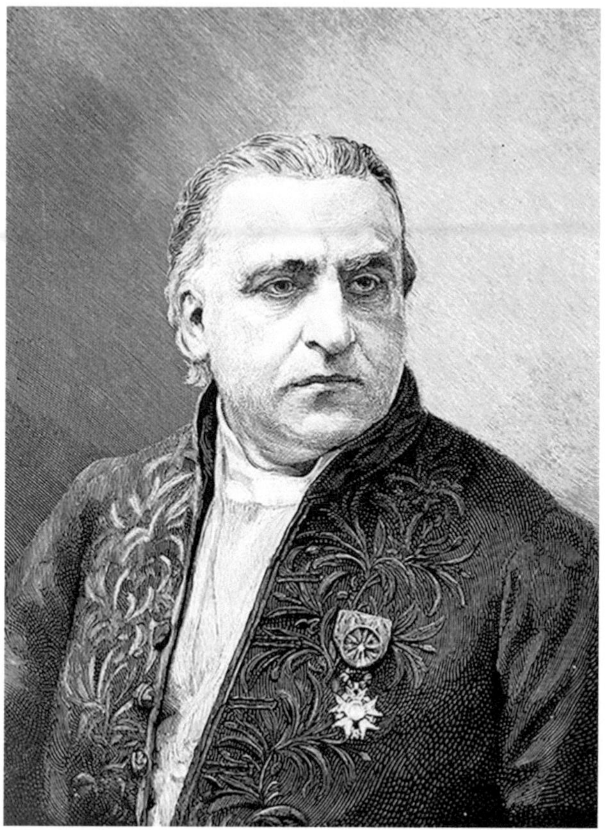

comprehensive neurological examinations, exemplifies his mastery of observation and deduction. His methodological legacy continues to inspire successive generations of medical professionals, who build upon his foundational contributions to advance the field of medicine.

Further Reading

Brigo F, Zanchin G, Martini M, Lorusso L, Study Group on the History of Neurology of the Italian Neurological Society. Jean-Martin Charcot (1825–1893) and the "Alice in wonderland syndrome". Neurol Sci. 2022;43(3):2141–4.

Charcot J-M. Leçons du mardi. Paris: Bureaux du Progrès Médical; 1887–1888, 1888–1889.

Goetz CG. Charcot, the clinician: the Tuesday lessons. New York: Raven Press; 1987.

Goetz CG, Bonduelle M, Gelfand T. Charcot: constructing neurology. New York: Oxford University Press; 1995.

I Can't Believe My Eyes (And Actually I Should Not)! Don't Get Confounded by Confounders!

2

> *Later on, you will discover that one must not mistake the shadow for the prey.*
>
> —Jean-Martin Charcot, *Leçons du Mardi à la Salpêtrière*,
> November 15, 1887

> *The onset time of facial paralysis having been established, it is necessary to investigate whether there was a specific cause that could explain the sudden onset of the disease. In such cases, exposure to cold is commonly implicated in the majority of instances. Indeed, it appears certain, at least in many cases, that this etiology is quite real. For instance, on the day the [facial] paralysis appeared, our young man traveled by train from Paris to Boulogne-sur-Seine. However, it is highly improbable that he was continuously exposed to local cold throughout the journey. In fact, he was seated in the front seat, shielded from the wind, between two individuals who provided some protection against drafts.*
>
> —Jean-Martin Charcot, *Leçons du Mardi à la Salpêtrière*,
> June 19, 1888

Every day, we tend to believe that what appears in front of our eyes is certainly and undoubtedly true.

Thankfully, this is mostly (but not always!) the case. A good physician should always consider the possibility that what seems real is actually a mirage. Hormone replacement therapy reduces the risk of vascular disease, and women with breast cancer undergoing primary surgery survive longer than those receiving primary

F. Brigo, *Charcot's Lesson*, Neurocultural Health and Wellbeing,
https://doi.org/10.1007/978-3-031-71221-0_2

endocrine treatment. Exposure to cold weather leads to peripheral facial palsy (as in the case described by Charcot). Drinking coffee increases mortality. Eating lobsters leads to a longer life expectancy, and eating ice creams results in sunburns. All these associations are real. The problem is that, despite being real, they are also false.

These scenarios describe an association between two things, where one appears to lead to the other. If this association is indeed real, why should it be false? Unfortunately, not everything that is real is necessarily true. X can be linked to Y (so that whenever X is present, Y is also likely to be there), but this does not inevitably mean that X caused Y. There may be a third actor, hidden behind the scenes, responsible for what occurs on the stage. This invisible factor is called a confounder, and it is the real explanation for what we observe.

Consider the association between eating lobsters and living longer (Fig. 2.1). Is there anything that could explain this finding? Lobsters are notoriously expensive, and only wealthy people can afford to eat them regularly. Being rich is associated with both eating lobsters and living longer (for various reasons, including a healthier lifestyle). Wealth is the confounding factor that acts as the true cause for longer life expectancy among lobster eaters (and, incidentally, also among oyster eaters and champagne drinkers!). Conversely, both eating lobsters and living longer are effects of being wealthy. Similarly, drinking coffee increases mortality not because coffee causes mortality but because heavy smokers tend to also drink coffee and have higher mortality rates. Smoking is the confounding factor and, hence, the hidden cause of increased mortality among coffee drinkers. Thus, the confounding variable distorts the association between two phenomena by creating a non-causal link.

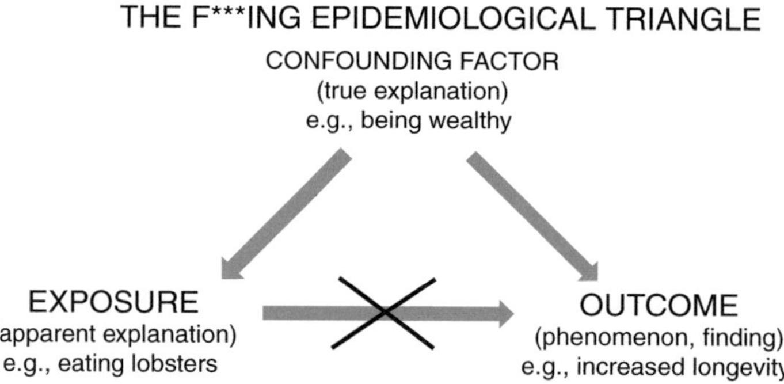

Fig. 2.1 The association between eating lobsters and increased longevity is misleading and false. This apparent association is actually due to a third factor: wealth. Wealth is correlated with both lobster consumption (exposure) and longevity (outcome), making it the true underlying explanation for both (confounding factor). These three factors—exposure, outcome, and confounding factor—form what is often referred to as the "eternal epidemiological triangle." Identifying and addressing these components in clinical studies and practice is the nightmare (but also the fun) of researchers and physicians. Given this complexity, it could also be called... "the f***ing epidemiological triangle"!

Sometimes, as in the case of ice creams leading to sunburns, the true underlying cause and explanation of the confounded association are obvious (in this case, sunny weather). However, in most clinical scenarios, the truth remains hidden beneath surface appearances.

Take for example the association between exposure to cold weather and the development of peripheral facial palsy. Many patients report this association, yet the most common cause of facial palsy is the activation of the *Herpes simplex* virus, which can be favored by cold weather but not caused by it. Before the role of viral infection was understood, all cases of facial palsy were attributed to cold weather (paralysis *a frigore*), which was a real yet false assumption. The same misconception applied to the association between cold weather and the flu or common cold. It took time to realize that the actual cause was not the most obvious *phenomenon* (a term derived from ancient Greek meaning "something that appears") but rather something concealed beneath the surface. What is essential is invisible to the eye.

Therefore, we cannot always trust our eyes and rely solely on what we see. But does this not contradict the fundamental essence of medicine, which is rooted in the observation of reality? What role, then, does clinical experience play in medicine?

What to Expect from Experience?

3

I have often said to you, it is better to observe than to read. Reading is good, but observing is even better; in just fifteen minutes spent observing patients, we can learn far more than from studying descriptions of their ailments in books.

—Jean-Martin Charcot, *Leçons du Mardi à la Salpêtrière,*
March 13, 1888

The concept of ex cathedra lessons is somewhat artificial. Relying solely on such teachings could leave you particularly vulnerable and prone to making serious errors when facing a patient.

—Jean-Martin Charcot, *Leçons du Mardi à la Salpêtrière,*
November 15, 1887

You know that my principle is to disregard theory and set aside all prejudices: if you want to see clarity, you must take things as they are.

—Jean-Martin Charcot, *Leçons du Mardi à la Salpêtrière,*
February 7, 1888

No doubt about it: experience is the cornerstone of medicine. Remove it, and the whole structure collapses. Spending time with patients is undoubtedly more rewarding and effective than reading books about them. However, we must recognize that, while crucial in clinical practice, experience alone is not infallible. I am not undermining the fundamental value of the experience accumulated over years of clinical practice. I am simply emphasizing its true significance.

F. Brigo, *Charcot's Lesson*, Neurocultural Health and Wellbeing,
https://doi.org/10.1007/978-3-031-71221-0_3

The ancients cautioned us wisely: "Life is short, and the art long, opportunity fleeting, experimentations perilous, and judgment difficult." Our clinical experience exposes us to only a limited aspect of the vast and complex landscape of disease. We do not encounter diseases directly; rather, we encounter diseases *embodied* in patients. What we observe reflects an intricate interplay between specific diseases and individual patients, influenced by numerous factors (age, sex, preexisting conditions, genetic factors, comorbidities, medications, disease severity, etc.). This complexity explains why each case in our clinical practice is unique and individual. It does not mean that there are no commonalities among patients with the same disease; rather, it highlights the limited and partial nature of knowledge derived from specific cases.

Moreover, the notion of "taking things as they are" to "see clearly," as recommended by Charcot, is not always straightforward (and the concept of confounding reminds us of this). For centuries, people observed that heavier objects seemed to fall to the ground faster than lighter ones, leading to the belief that weight directly influences fall speed. However, Galileo eventually disproved this notion, demonstrating that in the absence of air resistance, all objects, regardless of weight, fall at the same rate due to gravity.

Adopting an inductive approach can be useful in developing a more abstract knowledge that focuses on commonalities rather than on peculiarities, which could be applied to other similar conditions. Inductive reasoning enables physicians to draw generalized conclusions from specific information derived from everyday clinical experiences. This is similar to what occurs in clinical studies, where we observe a limited sample of subjects and obtain certain results. However, these findings are not always reliable; their accuracy, or closeness to truth, hinges on the study's methodological quality (known as "internal validity"). Biased studies may produce unreliable results.

Moreover, findings from studies involving a limited number of cases inherently possess some degree of imprecision. This stems from the fact that a clinical study typically focuses on a subset of patients rather than on an entire population (this can occur also for practical reasons. For example, studying all adults with epilepsy would be impractical). Consequently, the characteristics of the study population may not perfectly reflect those of the broader population from which they are drawn. Furthermore, patients are inherently diverse; even those with the same disease severity and treatment regimen may respond differently due to biological variability.

Life is characterized by variability, and every living organism is composed of dynamic elements subject to fluctuation (variables). In contrast, constants are typically encountered in physics and mathematics rather than biology. Thus, every clinical experience is inherently incomplete and imprecise, representing only a fragment of a broader reality. As Charcot himself acknowledged, "But I will be the first to recognize that my experience in such matters is far too limited for me to be allowed to draw conclusions with complete confidence (Charcot, Leçons du Mardi à la Salpêtrière, June 19, 1888).

Furthermore, we often assume that reality speaks for itself, appearing incontrovertible and self-evident. However, this is only partly true. We do not directly experience reality; rather, we perceive it. Reality unfolds before us as a series of phenomena (a term derived from ancient Greek meaning "something that appears"), which require an observer to be perceived. Sound or color exists only insofar as there is an ear or eye (and, ultimately, a functioning brain) to detect it. Everything we experience is filtered through our senses and processed by our brains. Therefore, our experiences are inherently subjective, and any filter through which they pass can distort reality.

In our everyday clinical practice, certain cases may leave a lasting impression due to their unique characteristics. Cognitive biases, such as anchoring or confirmation bias, can cloud our judgment and distort our perception of reality (see Chap. 12). While it is beneficial to be aware of these biases and employ strategies to mitigate their effects, it is crucial to recognize that humans are imperfect perceivers and biased interpreters.

In this context, the statement attributed to the German philosopher Nietzsche seems particularly relevant: "there are no facts, only interpretations." This raises the question: What role does theory play in clinical practice?

The Theory Is Good, but That Doesn't Prevent Reality from Existing

4

It appears that hystero-epilepsy exists only in France, and I could even say, as it has been said at times, only at Salpêtrière, as if I had conjured it into existence through sheer willpower. It would indeed be a remarkable ability to create diseases at whim and fancy. However, in reality, I am merely the photographer: I document what I witness, and it is effortless for me to demonstrate that these phenomena occur not only at Salpêtrière.

—Jean-Martin Charcot, *Leçons du Mardi à la Salpêtrière*, February 7, 1888

Let us first note, I repeat, the facts as they are; the theory will come later.

—Jean-Martin Charcot, *Leçons du Mardi à la Salpêtrière*, June 26, 1888

This child has been experiencing these attacks for three years. The first occurred in the morning when he woke up. Immediately, we attributed this to fear; this is the theory. The human being is essentially a theoretician. Unfortunately, he often constructs his theories indiscriminately.

—Jean-Martin Charcot, *Leçons du Mardi à la Salpêtrière*, January 24, 1888

F. Brigo, *Charcot's Lesson*, Neurocultural Health and Wellbeing, https://doi.org/10.1007/978-3-031-71221-0_4

As we explored in the previous chapter, facts do not exist in isolation; they are always intertwined with interpretations. On this point, Charcot would likely have disagreed. He was a strong proponent of positivism, which views science as a collection of facts, each representing an absolute and undeniable truth waiting to be identified. If only things were that straightforward!

Human reason does not passively absorb information from the external world to merely develop explanatory theories and draw generalized conclusions. It actively shapes reality by imposing order and structure upon the chaotic array of phenomena. Inductive reasoning, derived from the ancient Latin term *in-ducere*, meaning "to lead into" or "to infer," is a synthetic process. Much like a gardener focuses on the overall arrangement of colors rather than the individual species of flowers and plants, inductive reasoning moves from specific instances to general principles, abstracting the concept of a "flower" from the diverse flowers directly observed. It highlights commonalities over differences and peculiarities. In patients, it perceives not just individuals (literally "indivisible subjects", from the Latin word *in-dividuus*) but also representations of an abstract idea of disease. A disease that manifests itself uniquely in each patient.

While inductive reasoning begins with individual patient experiences and extrapolates to the broader concept of disease, deductive reasoning applies this general concept back to specific cases. However, in this deductive process, an interpretative framework is applied to reality—one that is not purely based on experience but is heavily influenced by existing theories. Our perception of reality is profoundly shaped by the preconceived notions we bring to it.

With all due respect to Charcot, who stated that "theory is good, but that doesn't prevent reality from existing," reality exists precisely because we perceive and interpret it in specific ways. The way reality appears to us is inevitably linked to how our senses perceive and process it. We make sense of what we observe, as reality is shaped by the perspective of the observer. If Charcot is correct in comparing us to photographers of the world, we must remember that each photographer selects their own frame and imposes their vision on the world they observe.

Charcot strongly advocated for the theory of heredity and degeneration, frequently inquiring about his patients' family histories and emphasizing degeneration as a central explanation for observed pathologies [1]. However, the indiscriminate use of heredity to explain the occurrence of disorders ultimately proved ineffective, and the whole theory of degeneration was later disproven. Charcot also firmly believed in the existence of "hystero-epilepsy," a condition characterized by convulsions, contortions, fainting, and transient impairment of consciousness. It was eventually revealed that this condition was largely an iatrogenic artifact, a disease inadvertently created by the very doctors diagnosing it.

Yet, when reading transcripts of Charcot's lectures, one cannot help but wonder how such a great clinician and observer, so grounded in experience, could become biased in constructing theories that diverged so far from reality—theories that crumbled like a house of cards instead of standing firm like a palace, ultimately proving unsustainable. The possible explanation lies in the fact that sometimes a theory persists despite being flawed, exerting its influence on our understanding of reality. To explain is to clarify, to smooth out irregularities, to level mountains, and to fill valleys. This process is necessary, especially in the face of complex clinical scenarios, but it also involves simplifying reality. Every problem (and every patient is such) should be simplified but not oversimplified. Simplification is beneficial, but excessive simplification is not. The risk is that a theory-driven approach may cause reality to lose its three-dimensionality, stripping it of its complexity and depth.

Given that both experience and theory are fallible, what should we prioritize? Should we favor one over the other, or should we abandon both, acknowledging the inherent limitations of clinical practice? A balanced approach, one that integrates both experience and theory, is the most effective way to address and overcome their respective shortcomings. Recognizing the strengths and weaknesses of each enhances our understanding of how we think and act. By avoiding becoming slaves to either our senses or our theories, we can use both to construct a more nuanced and robust understanding of reality.

Reference

1. Walusinski O. The concepts of heredity and degeneration in the work of Jean-Martin Charcot. J Hist Neurosci. 2020;29(3):299–324.

Induction and Deduction: Taken in the Loop

5

> *There is an important characteristic that can be exploited, as you understand, for the diagnosis in doubtful cases. The paroxysmal nervous accidents in our young patient are consistent with the law.*
>
> —Jean-Martin Charcot, *Leçons du Mardi à la Salpêtrière,*
> *February 28, 1888*

5.1 Induction: A Good Start Is Half the Battle

Induction, a cornerstone of scientific inquiry, involves deriving general principles from specific observations or instances. The term originates from the Latin verb *inducere*, meaning "to lead in." In clinical methodology and medical contexts, induction allows physicians to formulate hypotheses and theories based on experience and observations. It is a fundamental part of the scientific method, enabling researchers to propose explanations and predictions.

Unlike deduction, which starts with a general statement and derives specific conclusions, induction begins with specific observations and formulates broader generalizations. For example, observing the sun rising in the east every day leads to the conclusion that the sun always rises in the east.

Drawing general conclusions from specific observations is a key component and a fundamental method of the empirical approach to scientific inquiry. By noting repeated patterns or regularities, inductive reasoning allows for the formulation of general principles or hypotheses. Furthermore, inductive conclusions are not certain but are considered likely based on the evidence available (probabilistic conclusions).

Empiricism and induction are closely related, with induction serving as a fundamental method within the empirical approach. Empiricism relies on sensory

F. Brigo, *Charcot's Lesson*, Neurocultural Health and Wellbeing, https://doi.org/10.1007/978-3-031-71221-0_5

experience as the foundation of knowledge, while induction provides a way to organize and interpret these experiences, allowing for the development of general principles and theories. Data collected through observation and experimentation are then interpreted by inductive reasoning, identifying patterns, drawing broader conclusions, and helping develop and refine theories that explain observed empirical data. As more observations are made and patterns are recognized, theories can be refined and expanded.

Both empiricism and induction emphasize the importance of evidence in forming knowledge. Inductive reasoning ensures that conclusions are grounded in observed evidence rather than preconceived notions or speculation. Together, empiricism and induction form a robust framework for scientific inquiry and evidence-based practice, ensuring that knowledge is rooted in observable reality and is systematically organized.

5.2   Deduction: Logic in Play

Unlike induction, which involves reasoning from specific observations to general principles, deduction is a method of reasoning that starts from general principles or premises and applies them to specific instances (Table 5.1). The word "deduction" comes from the Latin verb *deducere*, meaning "leading down" or "deriving." While induction is a bottom-up process, deduction follows a top-down approach. What is particularly fascinating about deduction is that if the premises are true and the reasoning is valid, the conclusions drawn are logically certain. Furthermore, deductive arguments often follow a syllogistic structure, with premises leading to a conclusion. Deductive reasoning and syllogisms permeate mathematics or geometry, as in the following example:

Table 5.1 Main features and differences between induction and deduction in clinical practice and research

Criterion	Induction	Deduction
Definition	Inferring general principles from specific cases	Applying general principles to specific cases
Foundation	Observations and empirical data	Established theories and rules
Primary use	Hypothesis generation	Hypothesis testing
Methodology	Collecting data from experience and cases, identifying patterns	Starting with a theory, applying it to cases
Strength	Discovering new insights and patterns	Ensuring consistency with established knowledge
Example application in clinical practice	Noticing a cluster of symptoms or observing patient responses and proposing a new condition or treatment	Diagnosing a condition using established criteria and guidelines
Role in research	Essential for exploratory studies and identifying new phenomena	Crucial for validating experimental results

– Premise: All squares are rectangles.
– Premise: This figure is a square.
– Conclusion: Therefore, this figure is a rectangle.

Deduction can also start from empirical observations rather than from axioms or abstract data. Consider, for instance, the following example:

– Premise: All human beings are mortal.
– Premise: Socrates is a human being.
– Conclusion: Therefore, Socrates is mortal.

Here, both premises were derived from empirical observations, thus using an inductive approach. Induction serves to provide deductive reasoning with initial premises. The validity of deductive reasoning depends, therefore, on the accuracy of its premises established through induction. Conclusions drawn through deduction are only as sound as the induction behind them. Hence, assessing the validity of premises and understanding why they may be flawed is crucial.

The validity of premises depends, first and foremost, on the comprehensiveness of the observations gathered to formulate them, which directly impacts their precision. Consider, for instance, the following deductive reasoning:

– Premise: All mammals have a placenta.
– Premise: Cats are mammals.
– Conclusion: Therefore, cats have a placenta.

This reasoning sounds plausible. But can we be certain it is correct? The validity of this deduction hinges on the methods of observation used. If observations show that cats, dogs, dolphins, and cows—all mammals—have a placenta, the premise gains in comprehensiveness, precision, and validity. However, observing even one mammalian species without a placenta would suffice to undermine the validity of the initial premise. This was precisely the case with the platypus (*Ornithorhynchus anatinus*). The discovery of these mammals without placentas challenged the conclusions drawn from deductive reasoning based on inductive data.

In science, truth is not static; it is only valid until contradicted. What holds true today may not necessarily hold true tomorrow—it is true only if it withstands critical scrutiny. Gathering additional data can suffice to disprove its validity.

Moreover, the validity of conclusions resulting from deductive reasoning depends not only on the comprehensiveness and precision of its premises but also on their accuracy.

Consider the following:

– Premise: Heavier objects fall to the ground earlier than lighter objects.
– Premise: A rock is heavier than a feather.
– Conclusion: Therefore, a rock falls to the ground earlier than a feather.

At first glance, this conclusion appears valid and aligns with our expectations and experiences. However, what about its premises? Is it truly accurate that heavier objects fall to the ground faster than lighter objects? Is this everyday experience actually true? Can we conclude that weight alone is responsible for the falling speed? This empirical observation was formulated into law by Aristotle until Galileo disproved it in the seventeenth century. One can easily verify this by simply placing a stone and a feather in two closed boxes of the same shape and weight and then dropping them to the ground. By isolating weight from other factors influencing falling speed (such as shape), one can conclude that the statement that heavier objects fall faster than lighter objects—though empirically and immediately observable—is inaccurate.

Thus, such a conclusion would reinforce an observation that is itself inaccurate, risking its generalization and elevation to the status of law—a law with low validity.

5.3   Conclusions

The entire process of clinical thinking integrates both induction and deduction. The former provides observations and data that are further elaborated by the latter, giving rise to new conclusions. However, both are strictly interdependent. How comprehensive (and hence precise) were the data (or the evidence) used to draw conclusions? How accurate (and hence free from bias and distortion) were the original premises? How logically sound was the process of deduction in deriving conclusions from observations? Addressing these questions would improve our awareness of how scientific knowledge is produced and used in the clinical field.

Balancing induction and deduction can be challenging as it relies upon rigorous data collection, a critical appraisal of evidence, and a continual reassessment of diagnostic and therapeutic decisions. They should be seen not as conflicting alternatives to clinical reasoning but rather as complementary approaches that, thanks to their synergistic relationship, can enhance clinical outcomes and patient care. Mastering the integration of induction and deduction in clinical reasoning equips healthcare professionals with a robust framework to navigate diagnostic uncertainties, optimize treatment plans, and contribute to ongoing advancements in medical practice.

Nothing but a Domino Effect: Is Causation Really That Simple? 6

> *However, one reason we doubted their syphilitic origin is the significant delay of ten or fifteen years between the appearance of the chancre and the onset of nervous symptoms. This extended period is indeed notable, but it precisely characterizes cerebrospinal syphilis.*
>
> *—Jean-Martin Charcot, Leçons du Mardi à la Salpêtrière, November 15, 1887*

We administer a certain treatment to patients, and they recover. What could be simpler? It is as straightforward as playing dominoes: push one tile, and the next one falls, and so on. If only clinical reality were that simple! While the concept of causality is intuitively graspable (after all, even a child understands that pressing a button on a remote control turns on the television), it proves far more challenging to apply in clinical practice.

Causality is fundamental in science, which aims to deepen understanding by investigating causal relationships between phenomena. The Latin sentence *scire per causas* (knowing through causes) encapsulates this pursuit. Science is not just a collection of facts; it is a method that involves hypothesizing, experimenting, and analyzing results to uncover the underlying causes.

In medicine, establishing causal links between events or phenomena is a systematic process. It requires evaluating various potential explanations for observed outcomes before definitively determining cause and effect.

Consider the earlier example. How can we be certain that the treatment directly caused the clinical improvement? What other explanations must we explore and rule out first?

F. Brigo, *Charcot's Lesson*, Neurocultural Health and Wellbeing, https://doi.org/10.1007/978-3-031-71221-0_6

1. *Chance*: Firstly, we must consider that our observations could be purely due to chance. Chance permeates everything and cannot be ignored, even if its likelihood varies (for instance, meeting a friend who lives in the same city while walking the dog is far more probable than winning one million euros in the lottery). In clinical trials, the role of chance can be quantified using statistical methods like p-values. However, in everyday clinical practice, this quantification is much more challenging. Even if unlikely, we should always entertain the possibility that our observations might be solely due to chance.

2. *Natural history of the disease*: Some diseases improve or resolve spontaneously, regardless of any treatment. For example, a common cold typically lasts about a week, and a migraine attack may resolve within hours. Therefore, when we observe clinical improvement after treatment, it is crucial to consider how the disease would have progressed if left untreated.

3. *Placebo effect*: Merely believing that something could be beneficial often leads to real benefits, regardless of its actual efficacy. This phenomenon is known as the placebo effect and is inherent to every intervention, even those that are genuinely effective. The placebo effect occurs when individuals experience real improvement after receiving an intervention they believe to be effective. This effect can be influenced by expectations and beliefs. In randomized controlled trials evaluating experimental interventions, researchers can quantify (and minimize) the placebo effect by using a placebo—a substance that has no therapeutic effect. Unlike a sugar pill (which can affect blood sugar levels), a placebo is completely inert and lacks any biological or clinical effect. Additionally, a placebo is designed to look, smell, and taste identical to the experimental intervention, ensuring that neither researchers nor participants can distinguish between the two. For example, if a clinical trial shows that 40% of participants who received the experimental drug reported improvement compared to 10% of those who received placebo, the difference (40% − 10% = 30%) represents the actual efficacy of the drug beyond the placebo effect (10%). When a patient reports feeling better after taking a medication, it is important to consider the potential influence of the placebo effect.

4. *Regression to the mean*: Regression to the mean is a statistical phenomenon where an extreme value of a variable is likely to be followed by a value closer to the average upon subsequent measurement. In medicine, this often occurs when a patient with an extreme variable value (such as high blood pressure) is remeasured and found to have a value closer to the population average. This can lead to the mistaken impression that a treatment caused the change, when in fact, it may be due to chance. During the course of a disease, patients commonly experience natural fluctuations in their symptoms. For example, consider a patient with uncontrolled epilepsy who seeks a new antiseizure medication during a period of increased seizure frequency (the "crest" of the wave). If the seizure frequency decreases after starting the new medication, this could simply reflect a return to the patient's usual seizure frequency (the "trough" of the wave) rather than true improvement from the treatment. Therefore, it is essential to consider whether regression to the mean has influenced the perceived effectiveness of a treatment,

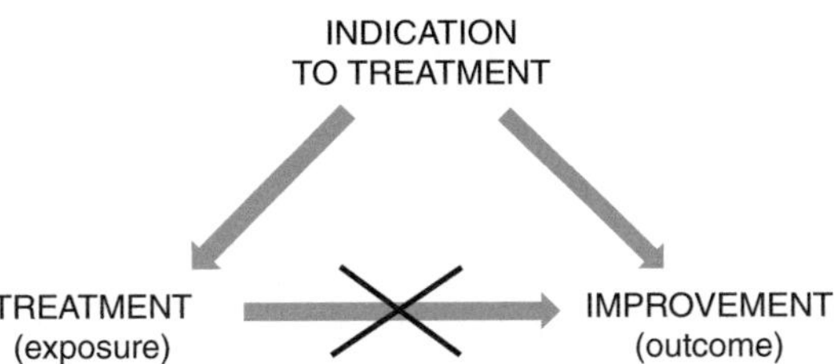

Fig. 6.1 Confounding by indication is inherent to medicine. The apparent association between a specific treatment and an outcome can often be attributed to a third factor: the physician's indication for treatment. Physicians prescribe what they consider the most appropriate treatment based on a patient's prognostic assessment. This indication can act as a confounding factor, influencing the observed outcome and complicating the interpretation of the treatment's true effect

as attributing natural symptom variation to an intervention could lead to erroneous conclusions.

5. *Confounding by indication*: This is a subtle confounding factor inherent in medical treatments (Fig. 6.1). Simply put, treatments are often given to patients whom physicians (consciously or unconsciously) believe are most likely to benefit. In other words, the observed efficacy of a treatment is not independent of the characteristics of the patients receiving it; rather, it is often tailored to those with specific prognostic factors. A study found that women with breast cancer who underwent primary surgery had longer survival rates than those treated with primary endocrine therapy. However, can we conclude that surgery causes longer survival in primary breast cancer? No. The choice of intervention was likely influenced by baseline differences in clinical and prognostic characteristics between the groups—for instance, differences in comorbidities, disease severity, or age. Therefore, the observed survival benefit might reflect these initial differences rather than the intrinsic effectiveness of the surgical intervention itself. Physicians routinely select treatment based on the clinical and prognostic characteristics of patients. This nonrandom selection process could lead to a spurious, noncausal association between the intervention and the outcome.

It is clear, therefore, that association does not imply causation. Similar to legal proceedings, we must first rule out all alternative explanations and possibilities before considering the hypothesis of a causal relationship—though this does not mean accepting it outright.

The question remains: What is the most appropriate and reliable method to investigate the causal relationship between two phenomena? How can we establish causality "beyond any reasonable doubt," similar to the legal standard of accumulating evidence to meet the burden of proof? Establishing a causal link is hindered by various factors, including selection bias (or confounding by indication) and chance. How can we minimize these obstacles? Surprisingly, the most effective way to mitigate these factors is by randomization—essentially, by flipping a coin.

6.1   Defeating Chance by Chance: The Miracle of Randomization

The most effective and reliable way to determine whether exposure to a particular intervention causes an outcome rather than just being associated with it is through experimentation. Randomized controlled trials (RCTs) are the study design that can provide the most robust evidence of a causal relationship between exposure to a medical treatment and a health outcome (Fig. 6.2).

Everything becomes clearer when framed in terms of comparisons. Day and night, sadness and joy, hot and cold—without a comparator, we would be lost in a world of uniformity where everything blurs together. As the old joke goes, "How's your wife?" "Compared to what?"—to truly understand reality, we need comparisons. In a randomized controlled trial, the inclusion of a control group allows us to estimate the net benefits in terms of effectiveness and/or tolerability that can be achieved by one intervention over another. When the comparator is an inert substance indistinguishable from the experimental intervention, it helps measure the placebo effect and isolates the true efficacy of the intervention.

So far, so good. But why should we ever rely on chance to establish whether a treatment is truly effective? In everyday clinical practice, no one flips a coin to decide whether to administer drug X or drug Y. The reason is that in a randomized controlled trial, randomization—or random allocation to the intervention or comparator—minimizes the effects of chance and confounding by indication, leading to

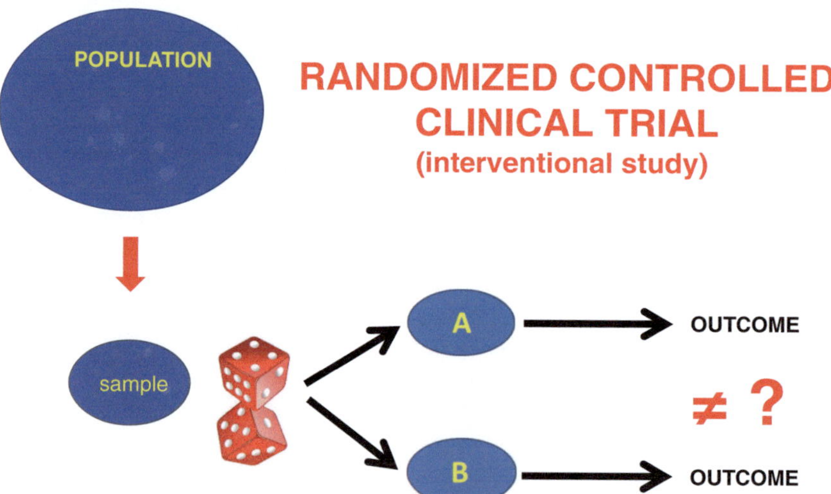

Fig. 6.2 A randomized controlled clinical trial is a scientific experiment designed to evaluate the effects of different interventions. A representative sample of patients is selected from the reference population based on prespecified inclusion and exclusion criteria. Participants are then randomly assigned to one or more intervention groups. These groups are followed over time to monitor differences in one or more prespecified outcomes. This process helps ensure that the observed effects are attributable to the interventions rather than other factors

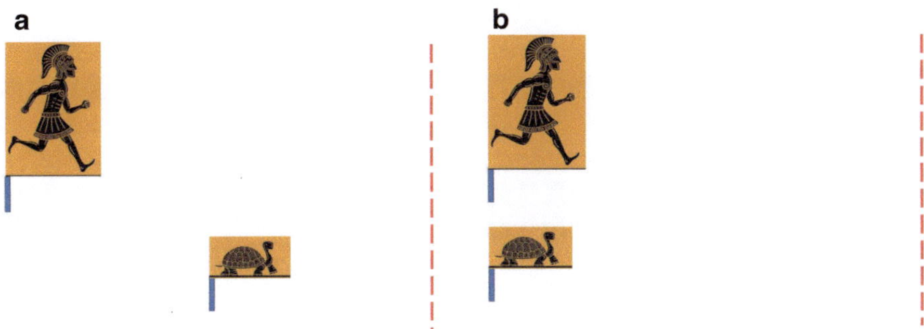

Fig. 6.3 Having two identical groups at baseline ensures that participants are placed under equal conditions, without favoring or disadvantaging anyone. A clinical study can be compared to a running race: in a nonrandomized controlled trial, the starting blocks are unevenly placed. In other words, there is an imbalance at baseline in factors that could influence the study outcome (**a**). In such a scenario, the slower turtle might cross the finish line ahead of the faster Achilles, leading to inaccurate results and biased conclusions. Conversely, if randomization effectively balances the prognostic characteristics of study groups at baseline, the starting blocks are aligned (**b**). This gives all participants an equal chance of winning, leading to more accurate and less biased conclusions

more reliable results regarding the causal association between exposure to the intervention or comparator and a specific outcome. Why is this so? The reason is that chance is the most democratic, inclusive, and unbiased force imaginable. Like the Roman goddess Fortuna (luck), chance is blindfolded: it does not play favorites, treats everyone equally, and gives everyone the same opportunities (Fig. 6.3). The probability—at least theoretically, and practically so in large samples—of getting heads or tails when flipping a coin is equal—50/50. By using a coin toss to assign participants to either the experimental intervention or the comparator, each person is given an equal chance of exposure. This equality of opportunity ensures that there are no differences, even in the characteristics of participants, between the two groups. If randomization has been effective, the two groups should be virtually identical at baseline in every respect—sex, blood pressure, income, shoe size, underwear size, political attitudes … everything! Importantly, effective randomization ensures that the groups are balanced in terms of clinical characteristics, including those that may influence prognosis or study outcomes (Fig. 6.4). But there's more! Effective randomization balances the groups not only in terms of known prognostic factors but also unknown ones (like potential future discoveries in genetic profiles). This is incredibly valuable. For example, if, in 100 years, it is discovered that underwear size affects blood pressure control (a plausible scenario, right?), the results of a well-conducted RCT comparing two antihypertensive treatments would still be valid because, from the start, the two groups were perfectly matched and comparable.

Hence, in randomized controlled trials, predictive factors (both known and unknown) tend to be balanced between intervention and comparison groups at baseline. The more similar these groups are, the more effective the randomization process has been. To assess the effectiveness of randomization in a trial, examine the table detailing the baseline characteristics of participants in each group. If no

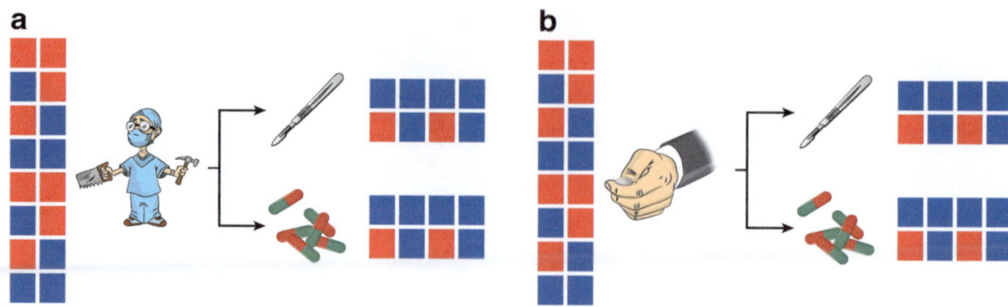

Fig. 6.4 In a controlled study without random allocation (**a**), the investigator decides which participants receive which interventions. Due to the inherent risk of confounding by indication, this assignment method does not prevent baseline differences in prognostic factors between groups. Such imbalances could influence the study results. For instance, if a surgeon assigns participants to either a surgical procedure or conservative medical treatment, more severe cases (represented by red squares) might receive medical treatment because they are not suitable candidates for surgery. In contrast (**b**), effective random allocation uses chance to create groups that are expected to be very similar—and theoretically identical—at baseline. Randomization helps produce comparable groups by balancing measured and unmeasured variables, known and unknown prognostic factors, and other participant characteristics. As a result, any differences in outcomes between the groups can be attributed to the interventions themselves, as this is the only difference between groups

differences are evident, it indicates that randomization has likely been effective in balancing known (and probably also unknown) variables.

The advantage of starting with identical groups at baseline is that comparisons can be made based solely on their exposure to the experimental intervention or comparator. If, upon completion, the randomized controlled trial reveals a difference between the experimental and control groups, this difference can be attributed to the intervention itself. This is because all other potential factors influencing the outcome were balanced at baseline, effectively minimizing their impact on the study results.

Thus, randomization mitigates confounding by indication and the effects of chance. Exposure is not assigned by investigators (which could introduce confounding by indication) but is determined purely by chance. Randomization isolates the intervention's effect, allowing it to be clearly distinguished from the background noise of confounding factors and chance. In this way, randomized controlled trials effectively explore and demonstrate the causal relationship between exposure to a specific intervention and outcome.

For example, observational studies initially suggested that hormone replacement therapy reduces the risk of vascular disease. However, when tested in a randomized controlled trial, this association was found to be false: hormone replacement therapy actually increases the risk of vascular disease compared to placebo.

6.2   Etiology and Causality

Randomized controlled trials are the most effective and reliable method for investigating and establishing the causal link between a treatment and a health outcome. However, when it comes to understanding the etiology of a disease, demonstrating causality can be more complex.

The philosopher Immanuel Kant (1724–1804) argued that the concept of cause and effect is an interpretative framework deeply embedded in our understanding reality. Therefore, different paradigms of causality can lead to varying conclusions about the causal relationships among phenomena.

There are two primary paradigms or models of causality. The first is the deterministic model of causality, which asserts a close, often direct, association between cause and effect. A cause can be necessary, meaning that without it, the disease cannot occur—such as *Mycobacterium tuberculosis* being necessary for tuberculosis. Alternatively, a cause can be sufficient, meaning its presence always leads to the disease, as seen in certain genetic disorders. Some causes can be both necessary and sufficient. This model an be visualized as an arrow, indicating a direct causal relationship from cause to effect.

The second paradigm is the probabilistic model of causality, which posits that a cause increases the probability of an effect occurring. In this paradigm, the cause is considered one of many contributing factors within a broader causal framework. Causality is akin to assigning a "weight" or score to each contributing factor. This approach is particularly relevant when multiple factors contribute to disease etiology, represented metaphorically as a puzzle made of pieces of varying sizes that together form the complete picture.

How then do we evaluate causal relationships in disease etiology or in everyday clinical practice more broadly? What criteria can guide our reasoning and inform our judgments on causality?

6.3   Criteria for Establishing Causation in Medicine

Given that association does not imply causation, we absolutely need reliable guidelines to define what causation is and how to recognize it. The criteria for establishing whether an association between two phenomena or events is also causal were proposed by Austin Bradford Hill (1897–1991), the founder of modern medical epidemiology, in 1965 [1]. Although there has been some debate about which criteria are the most crucial, they have been reiterated numerous times and remain valid.

Below, I present these criteria in an order I find most useful, though it differs from the original sequence:

1. *Temporal direction/sequence*: Before and after, not after and before. There is no doubt that in a causal relationship, the cause (antecedent) precedes the effect (consequent and … consequence!). Hence, to establish causality, we need to ascertain whether the exposure preceded the outcome. This seems straightfor-

ward, but sometimes it is easier said than done. For instance, cross-sectional studies cannot assess causality because they measure both exposure and outcome at the same point in time (a snapshot), making it impossible to determine which occurred first. Consider a study revealing that women with eating disorders often suffer from depression. What is the temporal sequence between the two? Which is the exposure, and which is the outcome? Which is the cause, and which is the effect? One might hypothesize that eating disorders cause depression, but the reverse (depression causing eating disorders) is equally plausible. This dilemma is akin to the famous chicken-or-egg causality problem.

While other criteria may or may not be fulfilled, this is perhaps the only one that always must be met to establish causation. Indeed, if X causes Y, X must precede Y in time. However, the reverse is not necessarily true: just because X precedes Y does not prove that X causes Y (this is known as the post hoc fallacy, derived from the Latin phrase "Post hoc ergo propter hoc," meaning "after this, therefore because of this"). Thus, the criterion of temporal sequence is necessary but not sufficient for establishing causation.

Furthermore, establishing a causal relationship can be particularly challenging if the effect occurs long after the exposure, as in the emblematic case of neurosyphilis, described by Charcot at the beginning of this chapter. The length of time between exposure and outcome reflects the pathophysiological mechanisms underlying the development of a specific disease and the complex interaction between causal agents and the patient.

2. *Strength of the association*: A tight connection! A causal relationship is a robust and direct association that can be likened to a taut string linking two objects. Similar to a taut string, a causal relationship is firmly bound and is resistant to breaking. The strength of this relationship hinges on how profoundly the cause influences the effect. Greater influence translates to a stronger causal relationship. The intensity of association is quantifiable through measures such as relative risk or odds ratio; higher values indicate a more potent link between exposure and outcome.

3. *Consistency of the association*: "One swallow does not make a summer!" A genuine association requires replicability, much like a true causal relationship. Multiple studies employing diverse methods to test the same causal hypothesis should yield consistent results.

4. *Biological gradient*: The greater the cause, the greater the effect. An increase in the exposure should result in a proportional increase in the outcome, demonstrating a clear dose-response relationship. For example, the more hamburgers you eat, the higher your LDL cholesterol increases.

5. *Specificity of association*: One exposure, one outcome. The idea here is that a causal relationship is often (though not always) specific, meaning a particular exposure leads to a specific outcome. For instance, drinking high amounts of beer can lead to liver cirrhosis, not the flu. However, one exposure can cause different and several outcomes. For example, alcohol can cause liver cirrhosis, polyneuropathy, and dementia.

6. *Biological plausibility*: Does it make sense? It refers to the biological mechanism that explains how the cause leads to the effect. In other words, it is the

plausibility of the relationship between the cause and the effect based on known biological facts. The more evidence there is to support the association between two phenomena in terms of biology, physiology, or pathophysiology, the more likely it is that one explains the other and possibly causes it. Biological plausibility is particularly crucial in disciplines such as ecology, toxicology, and carcinogenesis, where conducting experiments and directly observing effects can be challenging. While this criterion alone is not sufficient to prove causality, it remains an essential factor in epidemiological studies, especially in disciplines that inform public health decisions, preventive strategies, and safety standards.

7. *Coherence with existing knowledge*: Is it in line or misaligned? This criterion refers to the consistency of the causal relationship with what is already known about the natural history of the disease and other established facts. In other words, the causal relationship should align with existing theories, hypotheses, and knowledge.

8. *Experimental evidence*: Prove it to me! Randomized controlled trials could provide robust evidence for the causal association between exposure and outcome as this experimental design minimizes bias and confounding, leading to more accurate results. While experimental evidence is a crucial criterion for establishing causation, it is not always feasible or ethical to conduct experiments in humans. In such cases, other criteria such as consistency, plausibility, and coherence can be used to support the causal relationship.

9. *Analogy*: Is this like that? The use of analogies or similarities between the observed association and other known associations can be helpful in establishing a causal relationship. However, this criterion has its limitations and may not always be applicable. For instance, drugs may cause neonatal malformations with similar mechanisms to those observed with thalidomide in pregnancy.

6.4   The Long, Long Way to Causation

Establishing whether an association between two phenomena or events is truly causal requires navigating through a series of challenges, akin to passing through multiple doors. Unveiling the true nature of an association involves progressive elimination, much like Michelangelo freeing the figure from his marble blocks. Before concluding causation, we must meticulously consider and rule out confounding factors, systematic errors (biases), and chance occurrences (random errors). When confronted with any association encountered in clinical practice, we must ask ourselves: Is it spurious, merely reflecting chance or bias? If genuine, could it be influenced by confounding, where both phenomena are actually the effects of a third factor? If confounding is not an explanation for the observed association, how does each phenomenon fit into the chain of causal relationships?

Reference

1. Hill AB. The environment and disease: association or causation? Proc R Soc Med. 1965;58(5):295–300.

Let's Think About It! Metacognition of Clinical Thinking

> *This is something that should resonate with you and evoke anticipation of a specific diagnosis in your mind.*
>
> —*Jean-Martin Charcot, Leçons du Mardi à la Salpêtrière,*
> *May 1, 1888*

> *And it is precisely this combination of symptoms from two distinct conditions that can, at times, confuse the doctor, which makes the case interesting.*
>
> —*Jean-Martin Charcot, Leçons du Mardi à la Salpêtrière,*
> *June 12, 1888*

Clinical medicine is primarily a cognitive process, and understanding human cognition is crucial for improving our clinical thinking, enhancing diagnostic skills, recognizing and mitigating biases, and making sound decisions.

It has been said that human beings are the only animals capable of thinking. Whether this assertion holds true or not, humans certainly possess the ability to think about their own thinking. This process, known as metacognition, involves reflecting on one's own thinking processes, monitoring them, and regulating cognitive activities. Developing metacognitive skills enables clinicians to become more aware of their cognitive biases and errors, allowing them to take corrective measures.

According to the dominant dual-process theory of human cognition, cognitive processes involve two distinct systems. System 1 operates intuitively and unconsciously, relying on heuristics or mental shortcuts. It is the brain's fast, automatic, and intuitive mode of thinking that requires minimal effort and is used most frequently. System 1 generates intuitions that aid in performing tasks, although these intuitions are not always accurate. System 2, in contrast, represents conscious,

F. Brigo, *Charcot's Lesson*, Neurocultural Health and Wellbeing, https://doi.org/10.1007/978-3-031-71221-0_7

analytical thought. It operates slower than System 1 and involves a more deliberate, logical mode of thinking that requires significant effort. System 2 monitors System 1 and corrects it when necessary.

These two systems are like my sister and me: I tend to be impulsive and quick in decision-making (which, admittedly, can be risky, especially in matters involving love and women!), while she is analytical, cautious, and thoughtful (sometimes even a bit boring due to her thoroughness).

These models of thinking often lead to different conclusions. System 1 tends to jump to conclusions quickly sometimes based on incomplete information, whereas System 2 takes a more measured approach, considering all available information before making a decision. Heuristics, or mental shortcuts, are frequently used by System 1 to answer complex questions by substituting them with simpler ones. However, these heuristics can lead to cognitive biases, such as the halo effect, where individuals form a positive impression of someone based on a single positive trait. These cognitive biases can result in errors in judgment.

Both systems have strengths and weaknesses, and understanding their dynamics can aid in making informed decisions and avoiding cognitive biases (Table 7.1).

Table 7.1 Main features and differences between System 1 and System 2 thinking in clinical practice

Aspect	System 1 thinking	System 2 thinking
Nature	Intuitive, fast, automatic	Analytical, slow, deliberate
Decision-making process	Relies on heuristics and pattern recognition	Involves systematic reasoning and analysis
Speed	Rapid, often instantaneous	Time-consuming, requires more cognitive effort
Accuracy	Can be prone to errors due to biases and shortcuts	Generally more accurate but slower due to thoroughness
Situations	Best for routine, familiar situations	Best for complex, novel, or uncertain situations
Cognitive load	Low, minimal cognitive effort required	High, significant cognitive resources needed
Risk of error	Higher due to reliance on shortcuts and potential biases	Lower due to careful, deliberate analysis
Emotional influence	More susceptible to emotions and stress	Less influenced by emotions, more logical
Training and expertise	Utilizes tacit knowledge gained through experience	Requires formal education and conscious effort
Flexibility	Less adaptable to new information	More adaptable to new data and changing situations
Examples of use in clinical practice	Deciding on treatment for a well-known condition, making rapid triage decisions	Conducting a thorough review of a patient's history and test results, planning a complex medical intervention
	Quickly recognizing a common condition, diagnosing based on experience	Evaluating rare diseases, complex differential diagnoses

Usually, System 1 is often seen as the primary source of errors and biases, which is true. However, System 2 can also be ineffective. In clinical practice, each system can be prone to biases, especially when operating in isolation.

System 1, somewhat elusive, typically relies on pattern recognition, gestalt, and gut feeling. It can be highly efficient and reliable, especially with sufficient experience, but pattern recognition can fail for various reasons. Developing a pattern requires extensive experience to discern a consistent pattern amid diverse clinical presentations. Moreover, patients may not fit the classic disease pattern, leading to potential missed or incorrect diagnoses. Conversely, what appears as a classic pattern may not be the most prevalent in different populations as patterns evolve with changing demographics.

On the other hand, System 2, the analytical counterpart, excels in differential diagnoses, encompassing even the most subtle and rare conditions. Yet knowing every detail from medical textbooks does not ensure flawless execution in practical scenarios. Particularly in emergencies, the ability to quickly grasp the situation and initiate treatment based on expert heuristics is often more effective than consulting extensive literature.

Both systems function best when integrated, leveraging their strengths and offsetting weaknesses through coordinated efforts. System 1 should stimulate and inspire System 2, which acts as a supervisor and potential gatekeeper. Rather than opposing entities, they should be viewed as complementary components of human cognition. System 1 sparks initial hypotheses based on gestalt, gut feelings, and clinical experience. These hypotheses are then refined by System 2, which applies deeper epidemiological knowledge and analytical categorization of disease characteristics to solidify diagnoses.

Further Reading

Kahneman D. Thinking, fast and slow. New York: Macmillan; 2011.

The Razor That Does Not Split Hairs

8

> *It is therefore a well-established principle, and so I return once again to my favorite precept: do not multiply entities without necessity. You would never end it if varieties had to be the subject of completely childish classifications.*
>
> —Jean-Martin Charcot, *Leçons du Mardi à la Salpêtrière,*
> *December 20, 1887*

Occam's razor, one of Charcot's favorite precepts, is named after William of Ockham (or Occam; c. 1285–1347), a fourteenth-century English logician, scholastic philosopher, and Franciscan friar. The principle is also known as the "law of parsimony" or the "law of economy." The term "razor" refers to the idea of cutting away unnecessary assumptions or explanations.

The common formulation of this principle—though it does not appear in any of William of Ockham's surviving writings—is that "entities should not be multiplied beyond necessity" (in Latin, *entia non sunt multiplicanda praeter necessitatem*).

Occam's razor was not originally developed for medicine, but it has been widely adopted in the field as a guiding principle for diagnosis. It states that when a patient presents with multiple symptoms, the clinician should seek a single diagnosis rather than diagnosing multiple different ones. This principle is based on the idea that the simplest explanation is usually the correct one. In other words, the diagnosis that requires the fewest assumptions is the most likely.

In medicine, Occam's razor is often referred to as "diagnostic parsimony." This principle is particularly useful when a patient has a complex set of symptoms that could indicate multiple diseases. By focusing on a single diagnosis, clinicians can avoid unnecessary testing and treatment, which can be costly and time-consuming. For example, if a patient has a headache, fever, and rash, the clinician may diagnose

© The Author(s), under exclusive license to Springer Nature Switzerland AG 2024

F. Brigo, *Charcot's Lesson*, Neurocultural Health and Wellbeing, https://doi.org/10.1007/978-3-031-71221-0_8

meningitis, which could explain all three symptoms, rather than diagnosing three separate diseases.

However, it is important to note that Occam's razor is not universally applicable in every situation. Sometimes, multiple diseases can occur in a single patient. This scenario is reflected in Hickam's dictum, which serves as a counterargument to the use of Occam's razor in medical practice. While Occam's razor implies that diagnosticians should assume a single cause for multiple symptoms, one form of Hickam's dictum states: "A man can have as many diseases as he damn well pleases" [1]. The principle is attributed to an apocryphal physician named Hickam, possibly John Bamber Hickam [2]. When a patient presents with multiple symptoms, Hickam's dictum suggests that clinicians should consider multiple diagnoses and thoroughly investigate each one.

Occam's error, a cognitive bias, occurs when a physician incorrectly concludes that all of a patient's symptoms are explained by a single diagnosis, without considering the possibility of multiple underlying conditions (see Chap. 12). However, if a patient does have more than one disease, it is reasonable to consider multiple diagnoses to account for their symptoms. In such cases, the principle of parsimony still applies, as long as each diagnosis is considered based on evidence and necessity.

References

1. Miller WT. Letter from the editor: Occam versus Hickam. Semin Roentenol. 1998;33(3):213.
2. Mani N, Slevin N, Hudson A. What three wise men have to say about diagnosis. BMJ. 2011;343:d7769.

Useless and Yet So Useful: Why We Should Keep Visiting Our Patients

Please observe, gentlemen, primarily his gait and take note of the sound he makes as each step causes his feet to hit the floor successively.

—Jean-Martin Charcot, *Leçons du Mardi à la Salpêtrière,*
November 20, 1888

When evaluating the role of the physical examination from an evidence-based practice perspective, it is necessary to recognize that evidence-based practice integrates the best available research evidence with clinical expertise and patient values to make informed decisions about patient care. Despite its name, which emphasizes only one aspect—evidence—it originates from the intersection of three domains: the best evidence from the literature, the clinician's experience, and the patient's values and preferences. If one of these aspects is less robust, the other two tend to compensate dynamically. For example, if the best available research evidence is limited or of poor quality, the clinician's experience and the patient's perspective become even more important in guiding clinical decision-making.

When evaluating the role of physical examination, one must consider that even if the evidence supporting its validity is limited or of poor quality, clinical experience remains crucial.

Clinical experience refers to the knowledge and skills that clinicians acquire through their training, practice, and interactions with patients. It encompasses both technical skills, such as performing a physical examination, and non-technical skills, such as communication and decision-making. Analyzing the contribution of clinical experience from a scientific perspective requires a systematic approach that takes into account the complexity and variability of clinical practice.

F. Brigo, *Charcot's Lesson*, Neurocultural Health and Wellbeing,
https://doi.org/10.1007/978-3-031-71221-0_9

The figure of Charcot can help us better define the elusive role of experience in physical examination. Analyzing his method could be useful to better understand the contribution of clinical experience to physical examination, regardless of the diagnostic contributions provided by instrumental investigations resulting from technological development.

Upon the death of the French master, one of Charcot's most illustrious students, Sigmund Freud, described his working method with these words [1]:

> He was neither reflective nor a thinker, rather an artistically gifted nature or, as he himself said, a *visuel*, a visual person. As for his working method, here's what he told us. He used to carefully observe, over and over again, the things he didn't know, thus strengthening the impression he had drawn from them day after day, until their intimate meaning suddenly revealed itself to him. The apparent chaos of the continuous return of the same symptoms was then ordered before his eyes, and new clinical pictures emerged from it, characterized and defined by the constant grouping of certain symptoms. The limit cases, the 'types', could be delineated in all their completeness with the help of a special schematization, and starting from these types the vision extended over the long series of less evident cases, the *formes frustes*, which, starting from this or that characteristic sign of a given type, faded towards indeterminateness.
>
> This kind of intellectual work, in which no one could be his equal, Charcot called 'doing nosography' and he was proud of it. Not infrequently he was heard to say that the greatest satisfaction a man can experience consists in seeing something new, or rather, in recognizing its novelty, and in many of his observations he returned to this point and to the difficulties and usefulness of this 'seeing', wondering why, in medicine, men always and only see what they have, at one time, learned to see, and judging it marvelous that one can suddenly see as new (new pathological states) conditions that are probably as old as humanity. And here he himself felt obliged to confess that he now saw, in his wards, something that had gone unnoticed for thirty years.

From Charcot's work emerges a systematic ability to impose order and structure on what might initially seem like a disordered and shapeless reality. This ability, honed through experience, allows for the identification of specific disease patterns—clusters of signs and symptoms that illuminate diagnoses, much like constellations reveal their patterns in the night sky. This recognition is a form of cognition, knowledge acquired through experience. While Charcot's method might appear almost artistic, it is important to clarify that referring to medicine as an "art" can be misleading. It might suggest that medicine is solely the product of individual creativity and talent, reserved for a select few. However, this is not the case. The expression "ars longa, vita brevis" from the Hippocratic aphorism is often misunderstood; the Greek term *tèchne* actually refers to practical, almost artisanal knowledge, gained through experience and continuous learning. That cannot be learned, and that conducting a precise medical examination is an esoteric activity reserved for a select few. Not at all! Anyone referring to the medical "art" by citing the Hippocratic aphorism "ars longa, vita brevis" forgets that the original Greek term used is the initial diagnostic probability by considering the epidemiology of diseases and the informative potential of diagnostic tests used. Therefore, physical examination is not merely an art but a rigorous science that embodies the essence of the epistemological process, understanding that knowledge is a continuous journey towards truth rather than a final destination—an asymptotic approach to truth.

From this perspective, history taking and physical examination represent the essential and invaluable starting point of the entire diagnostic process—the foundation and precondition of its validity.

Reference

1. Freud S. Charcot. In: Gesammelte Werke, I. London: Imago; 1952. p. 21–35.

This is a significant gap. As you move forward, you delve deeper into the diagnosis. You first notice a difficulty in speaking that, if you have a trained ear, will already provide some information. Secondly, you observe trembling of the lips, then trembling of the hands, difficulty in writing, spelling mistakes, omission of certain syllables, missing words, and large gaps in memory.

—Jean-Martin Charcot, Leçons du Mardi à la Salpêtrière, January 10, 1888

Let us therefore study our patient with the aim of verifying the proposed hypothesis. Along the way, we will certainly gather a number of additional arguments, beyond those we have already noted, that support its legitimacy.

—Jean-Martin Charcot, Leçons du Mardi à la Salpêtrière, July 10, 1888

Making a diagnosis is the result of a stepwise process. It is a complex activity that unfolds over time and involves the patient, the physician, and other healthcare professionals. It can be compared to an investigative process requiring the collection of several pieces of information to get a broader and more meaningful picture of the patient's health issue.

Although in everyday clinical practice the diagnostic process is not always straightforward, its underlying principles are linear and, to some extent, easy to understand and follow. The fundamental concept of diagnosis begins with an unclear situation. By systematically gathering relevant information, we gradually resolve uncertainties, moving from ambiguity to clarity, ultimately defining what was initially unknown.

The diagnostic process means refining probability. The main goal is to move from a low level of probability (diagnostic uncertainty) to a higher one, increasing confidence in the suspected diagnosis. However, an equally effective diagnostic process can begin with a certain level of probability and end with a much lower one. In the first case, we confirm a diagnostic suspicion, while in the second, we exclude it. Despite these different outcomes, the trajectory remains linear, always progressing toward a final probability that differs from the initial one. A successful diagnostic process is one that shifts the initial probability—either by increasing or decreasing it. Diagnosis is not only about identifying a specific condition but also about ruling out other conditions that may present similarly but differ in nature. In this sense, every diagnosis is inherently a differential diagnosis.

How is such a refinement of probability achieved? It is attained by performing a diagnostic test.

10.1   Bayes's Theorem: Will the Sun Rise Tomorrow?

Refining probability relies on Bayes' theorem and conditional probability. Don't be afraid—it sounds a lot scarier than it actually is.

Bayes' theorem describes the change in the probability of a given hypothesis based on new information. What is the probability of being struck by lightning? The unconditional probability is approximately 1 in 1,000,000 per year and 1 in 10,000 over a lifetime, regardless of the circumstances. However, you do not have to be a gambler to immediately understand that this does not apply if you are out running a few kilometers from home and a thunderstorm suddenly appears. Conditional probability is a measure of the probability that an event occurs given that another event has also occurred. The conditional probability of being struck by lightning depends on (or is conditioned by) whether there is a storm. When evaluating the chance of a certain event, always ask yourself: Is this probability influenced or dependent upon what one knows? Does an additional piece of information or evidence change our probability estimate? If so, you are dealing with a case of conditional probability.

The analogy of the Platonic man, who has been confined in a dark cave since he was born. One day, he breaks free and witnesses the sunrise for the first time. It's a breathtaking experience! However, as he watches the sunset later that evening with the cave woman, he is gripped by a nagging doubt: Was this sunrise a one-time event? Will it happen again tomorrow? Over the following days, after seeing the sun rise repeatedly, his confidence grows that it will rise again tomorrow. By continuously adding new pieces of evidence to his initial uncertainty, the caveman refines his predictions, making them more precise. Eventually, he becomes so certain that the sun will rise every day that he takes it for granted. Yet, despite this growing confidence, there's always a minuscule chance that one day the sun might not rise. However, such a probability (already small due to sunrise experiences accumulated over hundreds of thousands of years) is getting smaller and smaller so that it can be approximated to zero. How reassuring! This example illustrates how probability can increase with accumulating evidence, but rarely, if ever, reaches absolute certainty.

THE DIAGNOSTIC PROCESS

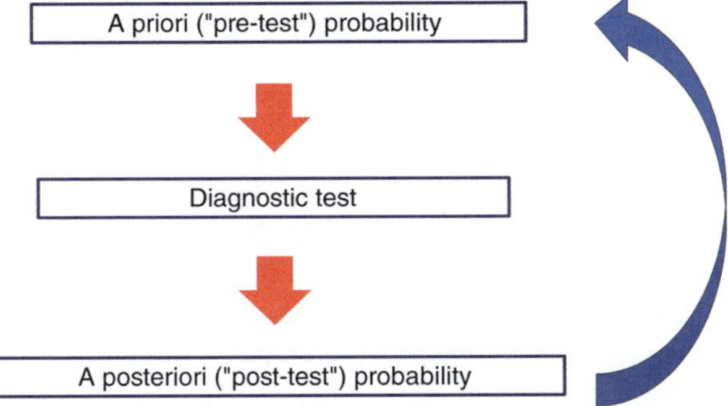

Fig. 10.1 The diagnostic process starts with a certain pretest probability and, after the application of a diagnostic test, arrives at a posttest probability of disease. This posttest probability can be sufficiently high to make a diagnosis or serve as a further starting point for applying additional diagnostic tests to refine the diagnostic probability. Like the hermeneutic circle proposed by the philosopher Hans-Georg Gadamer (1900–2002), it is an iterative process where initial probabilities (pretest) are refined by new data (test results), leading to updated probabilities (posttest)

Bayes' theorem is based on the idea that the probability of a disease is not fixed but depends on the probability of the symptoms and test results given the disease. In other words, the probability of an event depends on new information applied to what is previously known about the event. This concept can be simplified to the following equation: what we thought before (pretest probability) + test information (likelihood ratios) = what we think after (posttest probability). In clinical practice, we start with a certain pretest probability, and after the application of a diagnostic test, we finish with a posttest probability of disease (Fig. 10.1). Estimates of the likelihood of a disease range in probability on a scale from 0% (disease ruled out) to 100% (disease ruled in).

10.2 Pretest Probability

The pretest probability, or a priori probability, is the likelihood that a patient has a particular condition before any diagnostic tests are conducted. It serves as the starting point of the entire diagnostic process.

Several factors influence pretest probability. It can be estimated based on the patient's symptoms, medical history, and other relevant factors. Adequate knowledge of the epidemiological features of the disease (e.g., its prevalence, incidence, geographic and temporal distribution) is crucial for establishing an accurate pretest probability. For instance, hearing hoofbeats in the night would make you think of different animals depending on your location: a zebra if you're in the African savannah, or a reindeer if you're in Norway.

However, it is undeniable that the physician's "gut feeling"—a difficult-to-define mix of clinical experience, probabilistic reasoning (i.e., thinking in terms of how likely a certain condition is), epidemiological knowledge, and "good sense"—plays a major role in estimating pretest probability. Hearing hoofbeats with his eyes closed, the skilled physician thinks of zebras in Africa, horses in Central Europe, and reindeer in Norway. A less experienced one might think of zebras in Norway or reindeer in Africa—and the worst would think of dolphins in all cases.

When pretest probability is very high, further testing may be unnecessary. If the clinical picture is clear and testing won't add meaningful information, it's worth questioning the need for it. Conversely, when the pretest probability is extremely low, conducting tests also loses value. Diagnostic testing is most useful when there is genuine uncertainty, such as when two conditions are equally likely. Buridan's donkey was in the same situation: being equally hungry and thirsty, he was placed precisely midway between a stack of hay and a pail of water, stuck between two equally tempting choices. If only he had had a good test to shake his initial uncertainty!

Though it's not always possible to precisely quantify pretest probability, it's helpful to think in terms of likelihood. On a scale of 0–10, how confident are you that a patient has a particular condition? How much would you bet on your diagnostic suspicion? If your confidence is low, further testing is warranted to refine the probability.

Correctly estimating the pretest probability is essential as it shapes the entire diagnostic process. Just as buttoning the first button incorrectly misaligns the rest, a misjudged pretest probability can lead to diagnostic errors throughout the process.

10.3   Diagnostic Test

A diagnostic test is any tool or method that can alter the initial probability of a diagnosis. It doesn't have to be a blood test or imaging study; even a detailed medical history or physical examination qualifies as a diagnostic test if it helps refine the probability of a condition. A good diagnostic test is one that meaningfully shifts the pretest probability—either increasing or decreasing it. The more it changes the probability, the more valuable the test. A test that fails to modify pretest probability provides no useful information and is, therefore, ineffective.

Choosing the right test is crucial as it connects pretest and posttest probabilities. Before ordering any diagnostic test, the physician must understand its potential to provide meaningful information. The ideal test should be both accurate and precise (Fig. 10.2). Although sometimes used as synonyms, they are not. Accuracy refers to the ability to represent reality exactly as it is. An accurate test correctly identifies a condition—calling a rose a rose. An inaccurate test misidentifies conditions—calling a rose a daisy. Conversely, precision refers to the level of detail and resolution a test offers. A precise test gives a clear, focused picture of the situation, while an

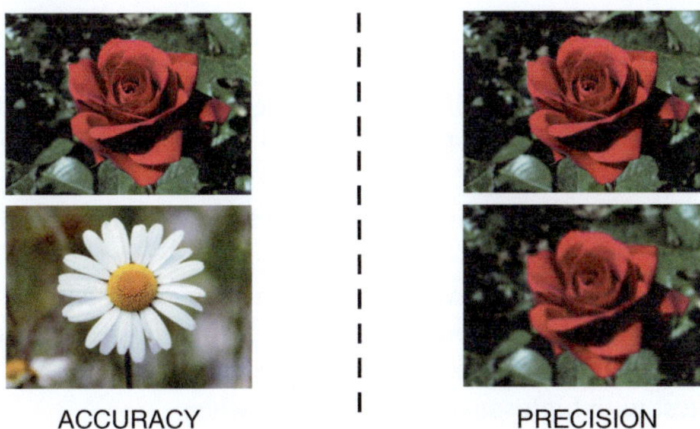

Fig. 10.2 Accuracy refers to a diagnostic test's ability to correctly represent reality. An accurate test identifies a rose as a rose, while an inaccurate one might mistake it for a daisy. Precision, in contrast, concerns the level of detail and focus a test provides. A precise test offers a clear, high-resolution picture of reality, whereas an imprecise test yields a blurry and indistinct image. Ideally, a diagnostic test should be both accurate and precise to ensure it provides reliable and detailed information about a patient's condition

imprecise test produces a blurry, vague image. While the best tests are both accurate and precise, if forced to choose one characteristic over the other, which would be more important?

Precision is not the same as accuracy. A test could be highly precise—yielding consistent results each time it is applied—but if it lacks accuracy, those results will be consistently wrong or far from the true value. Conversely, a highly accurate test, even if less precise, will provide results that are close to the truth, though they may vary slightly. Between the two, a more accurate test is generally preferable because it brings you closer to the true diagnosis, even if the results are not always identical. Precision, without accuracy, only ensures consistent but incorrect results, leading you down the wrong path repeatedly. A good diagnostic test should guide you toward the truth, even if the journey is not perfectly precise.

An accurate test is one that can correctly classify individuals according to their true health status. Ideally, all patients would be identified as such (true positives), and all healthy individuals would be recognized as healthy (true negatives). However, in practice, diagnostic tests are rarely perfect. A patient misclassified as healthy is termed a false negative, and a healthy individual incorrectly identified as sick is called a false positive. The best tests minimize both false positives and false negatives, ensuring most individuals are correctly classified as true positives or true negatives.

Accuracy, in this context, encompsses two important diagnostic parameters: sensitivity and specificity.

10.3.1 Sensitivity

Sensitivity is defined as the probability that the test is positive if the subject is affected by a disease (Fig. 10.3). It measures the test's ability to detect the disease when it is present, thus avoiding false negatives. When a test is maximally sensitive (sensitivity = 100%), it correctly identifies individuals who truly have the condition (true positives).

With a test that is 100% sensitive, if a person has the disease in question, the test will definitely be positive. Furthermore, among those who test negative, there are only healthy subjects (because the rate of false negatives is zero).

Choosing a test with high sensitivity is crucial when:

- The consequences of missing a true positive are severe (e.g., a life-threatening disease).
- The treatment for the condition is highly effective and has minimal side effects.

Furthermore, a sensitive test ensures that true positives are not overlooked, leading to timely intervention. For example, consider a diagnostic test for early-stage breast cancer. A highly sensitive test would accurately identify most women with breast cancer, reducing the risk of false negatives.

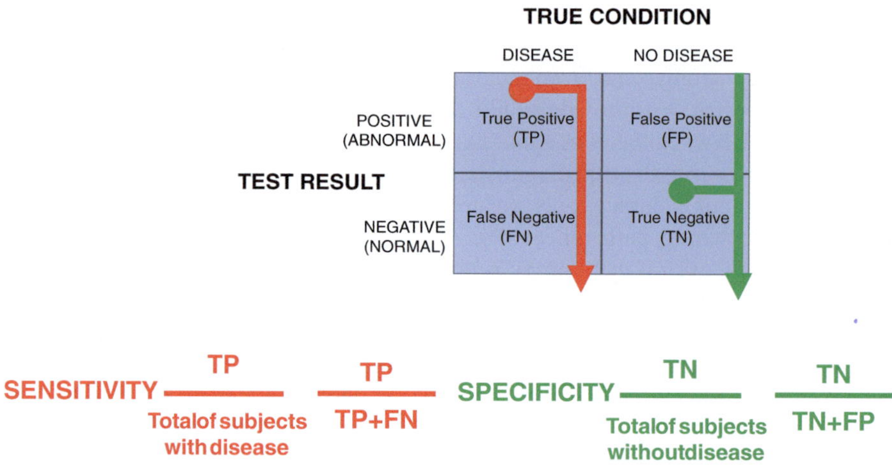

Fig. 10.3 The sensitivity of a diagnostic test measures its ability to accurately identify individuals who have the disease or condition of interest, indicating the test's capability to detect true-positive cases among all individuals who truly have the disease. It represents the proportion of individuals with the disease who test positive (or abnormal) on the diagnostic test. Conversely, the specificity of a diagnostic test assesses its ability to correctly identify individuals who do not have the disease or condition of interest. Specifically, specificity tells us how well the test can detect true-negative cases among all individuals who do not have the disease. It represents the proportion of individuals without the disease who test negative (or normal) on the diagnostic test

10.3.2 Specificity

Specificity is defined as the probability that the test is negative if the subject does not have the disease in question (Fig. 10.3). It measures the test's ability to correctly rule out the disease when it is truly absent, thereby avoiding false positives. When a test is maximally specific (specificity = 100%), it correctly identifies individuals without the condition (true negatives).

With a test that is 100% specific, if a person is healthy, the test will definitely be negative. Furthermore, among those who test positive, there are only patients (because the rate of false positives is zero).

Choosing a test with high specificity is crucial when:

– The consequences of false positives are significant (e.g., unnecessary treatments, anxiety, or stigma).
– The condition being tested for is rare or has specific implications.
– The test aims to definitively rule out the disease.

Furthermore, a specific test accurately excludes healthy individuals, minimizing false positives.

10.3.3 Sensitivity and Specificity: Pitfalls and Caveats

– Sensitivity and specificity are defined relative to a gold standard test assumed to be accurate. Using a different gold standard test as a reference would lead to changes in sensitivity and specificity.
– Specificity and sensitivity often involve a trade-off. Higher specificity may lead to lower sensitivity (more false negatives), but higher sensitivity may result in lower specificity (more false positives). Life is about choices and compromises.
– The rule of "SpIN-SnOUT": it is a test with high specificity (Sp) when positive (p) confirms the diagnosis (IN), whereas it is a test with high sensitivity (Sn) when negative (n) excludes the diagnosis (OUT).
– Achieving the right balance between sensitivity and specificity ensures optimal patient care, but it is important to consider your aim.
– Sensitivity and specificity depend on the test and not on the subject; they are independent of the prevalence of the disease!
– Diagnostic sensitivity can be likened to a watchful sentinel guarding against missed diagnoses. It empowers healthcare professionals to detect true positives and initiate timely interventions. Conversely, diagnostic specificity acts as a vigilant gatekeeper, ensuring that true negatives are correctly identified. It shields individuals from unnecessary interventions and guides clinical decision-making.

10.3.4 Likelihood Ratio

LR measures the test's ability to modify the pretest probability of disease (according to Bayes' theorem). Since a test can yield positive or negative results, there are two corresponding LR values:

- Positive likelihood ratio (LR+): it measures the information potential of the diagnostic test when it yields a positive result. It quantifies how much the probability of a person having the disease changes when the test result is positive.
- Negative likelihood ratio (LR−): it measures the information potential of the diagnostic test when it yields a negative result. It indicates how much the probability of a person having the disease changes when the test result is negative.

These ratios help us determine whether a test result significantly alters the probability that a specific condition (such as a disease) exists. They indicate how many times more (or fewer) a positive or negative test is found in patients compared to healthy subjects.

A high or low LR indicates that the test is valuable for a specific population as it significantly alters the posttest probability, increasing or decreasing it, respectively (Fig. 10.4). If the LR+ (for positive results) is greater than 1, the posttest probability

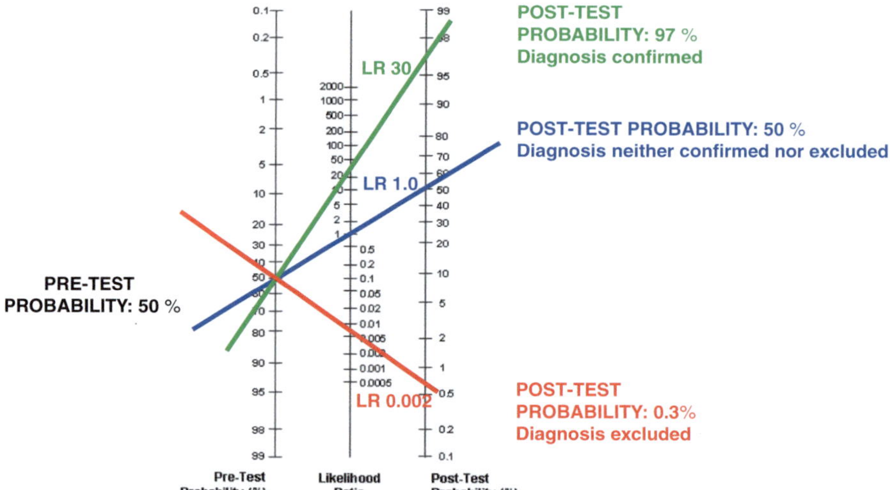

Fig. 10.4   If we begin with a pretest probability of 50%, we are essentially at a point of maximum uncertainty, similar to flipping a coin. This represents a state where the likelihood of a condition being present or absent is equally balanced. Now, if we apply a diagnostic test with a likelihood ratio (LR) of 1, it will have no impact on this uncertainty. The posttest probability will remain the same at 50%, making the test useless in refining the clinical suspicion. However, if we use a test with a high LR (e.g., 30), the posttest probability will significantly increase, greatly enhancing our confidence in the presence of the condition. This suggests that the test result strongly supports the initial suspicion and may allow us to confirm the diagnosis. Conversely, if we apply a test with a very low LR (e.g., 0.002), the posttest probability will drop drastically, indicating that the likelihood of the condition being present is now very small. This could lead us to reject the initial clinical suspicion, as the test result strongly favors the absence of the condition

of the disease being present increases, with higher values providing stronger evidence to confirm the diagnosis. Conversely, if the LR− (for negative results) is less than 1, the posttest probability of the disease being present decreases. Lower values of LR− provide stronger evidence to rule out the diagnosis. An LR of 1 means that the test is not informative and therefore not useful as the posttest probability will be equal to the pretest probability.

Likelihood ratios help determine whether a test result significantly changes the likelihood of disease presence, bridging the gap between test results and clinical decision-making. The larger the positive likelihood ratio, the greater the likelihood of disease; the smaller the negative likelihood ratio, the lesser the likelihood of disease. Likelihood ratios empower healthcare professionals to make informed choices, enhancing patient care and personalized medicine.

10.4 Posttest Probability

Posttest probability is the probability that the disease is present given the information available before the test and the test result. It is calculated using Bayes' theorem, which states that the probability of the disease given the symptoms and test results equals the product of the pretest probability and the likelihood ratio of the test. The relationship between pretest and posttest probability, mediated by the information provided by the diagnostic test, is visualized by a nomogram.

In the Bayesian approach to clinical diagnosis, the information obtained after performing the test adds to the pretest probability (what we thought before) and leads to the posttest probability (what we think after). If the result is informative, the test modifies the pretest probability. Otherwise, we are left with the same pretest probability. Diagnosis is a process that can vary in effectiveness, depending on movement, time, and resources used. Being stuck in quicksand due to an uninformative test is not ideal.

In some cases, the posttest probability is high enough to confirm the diagnosis or low enough to rule it out. If so, the diagnostic workup is conclusive as it has achieved its goal. Otherwise, the obtained posttest probability can serve as another starting point (or pretest probability) for further diagnostic evaluation through additional tests, leading to subsequent posttest probabilities. This process is dynamic and iterative, aiming to reach a final diagnosis.

10.5 Predictive Values

Sensitivity and specificity are critical diagnostic properties that reveal how well a test performs. Sensitivity measures the likelihood that the test will be positive if the subject has the disease, while specificity measures the likelihood that the test will be negative if the subject does not have the disease. Although these metrics are important for understanding a test's performance, they don't always answer the most pressing question in clinical practice: given a test result, what is the probability that the subject actually has or does not have the disease?

In everyday clinical scenarios, we often deal with cases where the disease status is uncertain. What we really need to know is the probability that a positive or negative test result reflects the true presence or absence of the disease. For example, if an axillary thermometer shows a body temperature of 38°C, we want to understand the likelihood that the patient actually has the flu. This practical information is more relevant to us than merely knowing how likely the test is to detect an increased temperature when the flu is present. What truly matters to us are the predictive values.

Positive predictive value (PPV) indicates the proportion of patients with positive test results who are correctly diagnosed (Fig. 10.5). It answers the question: If a patient tests positive, how confident can we be that the result truly reflects the presence of the disease? In other words, PPV helps us interpret the clinical significance of a positive test result, providing insight into the probability that the disease is actually present.

Negative predictive value (NPV) represents the proportion of patients with negative test results who are correctly diagnosed (Fig. 10.5). It informs us about the likelihood that a negative test result accurately rules out the disease. If a patient tests negative, how assured are we that they are truly disease-free?

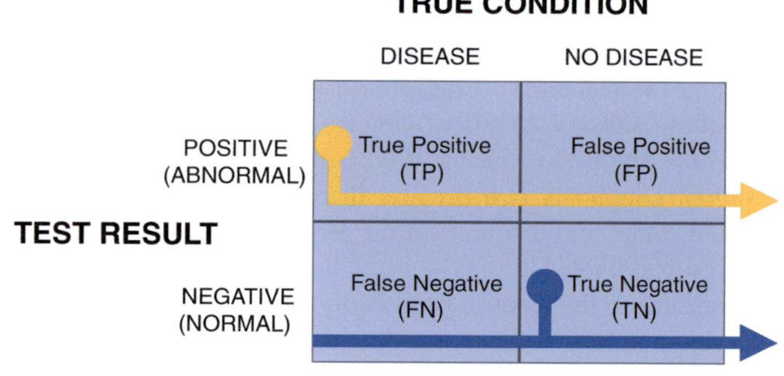

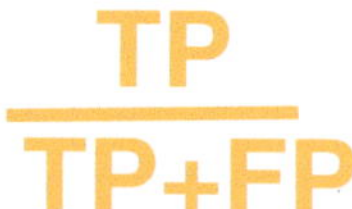

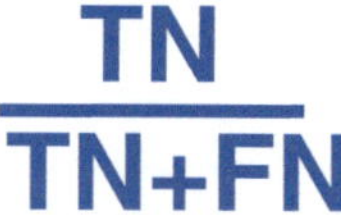

Fig. 10.5 Positive predictive value (PPV) is a statistical measure that assesses the probability that individuals with a positive test result truly have the disease or condition of interest. It represents the proportion of positive test results that are true positives, i.e., the test correctly identifies those who have the condition out of all individuals who tested positive. Negative predictive value (NPV) is a statistical measure that assesses the probability that individuals with a negative test result truly do not have the disease or condition of interest. It represents the proportion of negative test results that are true negatives, i.e., the test correctly identifies those who do not have the condition out of all individuals who tested negative

10.5.1   Predictive Values: Pitfalls and Caveats

- Predictive values depend on the sensitivity and specificity of the diagnostic test. If sensitivity increases (fewer false negatives), the negative predictive value also increases; if specificity increases (fewer false positives), the positive predictive value increases.
- Unlike sensitivity and specificity, predictive values depend not only on the test but also on the subject and, consequently, on the prevalence of the disease in the tested population (Fig. 10.6). Therefore, unlike sensitivity and specificity, which remain constant, predictive values can vary.
- As prevalence increases, the positive predictive value also increases. In other words, in a population where the disease is common, a positive test result is highly likely to correctly indicate the presence of the disease. However, as prevalence increases, the negative predictive value decreases. Thus, in a population where the disease is common, a negative test result is less likely to accurately indicate the absence of disease.
- If prevalence decreases, the positive predictive value also decreases, whereas the negative predictive value increases.
- Predictive values are crucial for linking diagnostic test results with clinical decision-making. They help interpret how test results relate to the likelihood of a disease, taking into account the prevalence of the condition in a given population. However, these values are not fixed or universally applicable; they vary based on the prevalence of the disease. For example, consider a body temperature of 38°C as a potential indicator of flu. The probability that this temperature signifies the flu depends significantly on the context in which the test is applied.

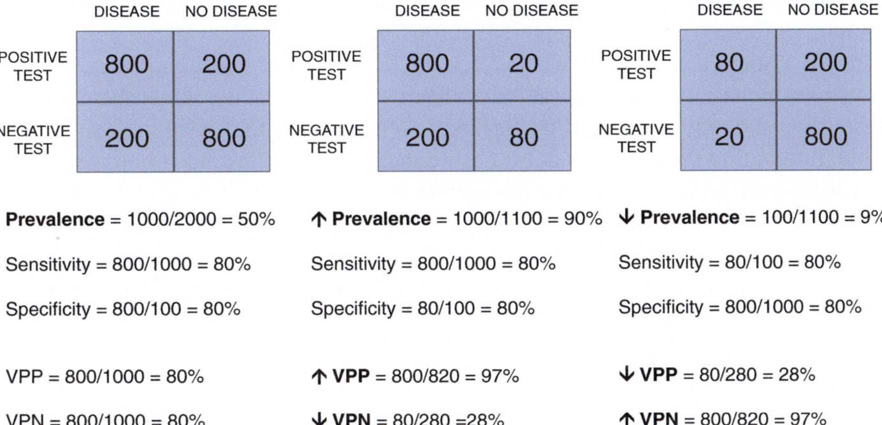

Fig. 10.6 Unlike sensitivity and specificity, predictive values depend not only on the test itself but also on the characteristics of the tested population, particularly the prevalence of the disease. Therefore, while sensitivity and specificity remain constant for a given test, predictive values can vary. When disease prevalence rises, the positive predictive value (PPV) increases, whereas the negative predictive value (NPV) decreases

This probability can change based on several factors. The likelihood of flu is higher in winter compared to summer. The probability differs if the test is performed in a kindergarten, where flu might be more common, versus an adult population with influenza vaccination. Furthermore, The prevalence of flu varies by region, so the probability would be different in Italy compared to Nigeria. Thus, interpreting predictive values requires considering the specific context in which the test is conducted, as these values are influenced by the prevalence and other situational factors.

10.6　Deciding Whether to Use a Test

Requesting a diagnostic test does not automatically mean that it should be performed. The decision to request or perform a diagnostic test is influenced by a complex interplay of clinical, patient-related, system-level, and contextual factors. Striking the right balance between early detection, patient preferences, and evidence-based practice is essential for providing optimal patient care. Several factors must be considered in this decision-making process. The characteristics of the test, such as its accuracy, sensitivity, specificity, and predictive values, play a crucial role in determining its utility. A test with high accuracy and predictive value is more likely to provide useful information. The prognosis of the disease also impacts the decision. The potential outcomes of the disease, including its natural progression and potential severity, influence whether a test is warranted. For instance, tests for diseases with poor prognosis might be prioritized differently compared to those for conditions with better outcomes. The availability and effectiveness of treatments are another important consideration. If effective interventions are available, earlier detection might be more valuable. Patient preferences must also be taken into account. Informed consent and patient autonomy should guide whether a test aligns with the patient's goals and wishes. Lastly, system-level considerations, such as resources including time, cost, and healthcare system capacity, affect the decision. Tests should be requested and performed in a manner that is sustainable and equitable. Integrating these factors helps ensure that diagnostic testing is both necessary and beneficial, enhancing the overall quality of patient care.

Not All Errors Are Created Equally: Biological Variability and Systematic Errors (Biases)

11

There is, however, one source of error that I will mention briefly, because I have encountered it at least once and couldn't avoid it.

—Jean-Martin Charcot, *Leçons du Mardi à la Salpêtrière, June 26, 1888*

While some arrows hit the target, not all of them strike the bullseye—unless you are as skilled as Robin Hood. Technically, arrows missing the bullseye can be categorized as errors, either major or minor, depending on their distance from the center. Some arrows are scattered randomly across the target, which is not surprising. Many factors influence their trajectory: the tension of the bow, the balance of the arrow, the archer's aim, visual acuity, concentration, wind direction, strength, and more. While some of these factors can be anticipated, many are unpredictable. Even with minimized variability, it is highly unlikely that any two shots will be identical (Fig. 11.1).

Now, consider a different scenario. You shoot your arrows, and they cluster together on the target, though far from the bullseye. This clustering suggests something more deliberate than random variation; it indicates a systematic force affecting the arrows' trajectories. For example, if your bow consistently veers arrows 30 degrees to the left, this systematic error would cause the arrows to group together, albeit away from the bullseye.

Not all errors are alike, and recognizing these differences can enhance your reasoning and help you avoid errors in clinical practice.

53

F. Brigo, *Charcot's Lesson*, Neurocultural Health and Wellbeing, https://doi.org/10.1007/978-3-031-71221-0_11

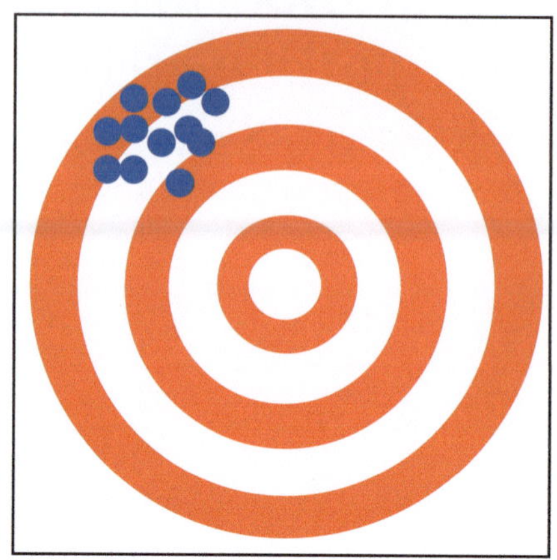

Fig. 11.1 This figure illustrates the concepts of sampling error and systematic error. The target represents the true value or population parameter we want to estimate. The dots represent individual sample estimates. In the first scenario (on the left), estimates are randomly scattered around the target. A sampling error occurs because each sample estimate is likely to differ from the true value due to random variation inherent in the sampling process. In the second scenario (on the right), sample estimates (dots) are clustered around a different point than the true value, creating a consistent bias away from the target. A systematic error arises due to flaws or biases in the measurement process or methodology, resulting in consistently inaccurate estimates that are consistently offset from the true value

One type of error arises from the inherent variability of biological processes. When measuring the same parameter repeatedly, slight differences in values are inevitable due to minor changes in the environment or measurement instruments. Biology is characterized by variability; life itself is dynamic and fluctuating. Each biological parameter represents a variable that fluctuates and varies within a defined range of values, unlike constants, which are more prevalent in the realm of physics.

This type of error is largely unavoidable as it is intrinsic to biological processes. However, its impact can be mitigated by conducting repeated measurements and observations. In clinical trials, the magnitude of this error can be quantified using confidence intervals that indicate the precision (or imprecision) of observed values. The width of these intervals depends on the sample size; larger samples yield narrower intervals, enhancing precision.

In nature, increasing observations brings us closer to the truth. For instance, a child who encounters a horse for the first time might mistakenly conclude that all horses are black. Only through repeated exposure to horses can one discern the true essence of "horseness" beyond the variability observed in individual horses. This realization aligns with Plato's idea that we live in a world where errors are inevitable, and the essence of truth is obscured by the diversity of life on earth.

The second type of error is far more insidious and severe than the first, although it can be predicted. Known as bias or systematic error, it systematically distorts observed values, consistently deviating from the truth. Despite their apparent precision, biased findings will inevitably be inaccurate or consistently different from the actual truth, much like arrows grouped closely but far from the target. The degree of inaccuracy (or the distance of an observed value from the true value) can be roughly estimated by the formula "inaccuracy = variability/bias^2". While variability contributes to inaccuracy, bias, being squared in the formula, has a more profound impact. Therefore, efforts should focus on preventing and mitigating systematic errors to preserve the accuracy and validity of observations.

Awareness of the main types of bias and their impact is crucial not only for those actively involved in clinical research but also for clinicians who interpret and apply the results of clinical studies. Below, I have listed the most relevant biases in clinical research to aid in critically appraising study results.

11.1 Biases That Can Occur in Interventional Studies

An interventional study compares the effects of two or more interventions or intervention strategies on a specific outcome across two or more groups of subjects. The classic example is a randomized controlled trial. To ensure the most accurate and unbiased results, the study groups should be as similar as possible. This similarity helps isolate the effect of the intervention from confounding factors, including the particularly insidious confounding by indication. The key issue is comparability. In an interventional study, the comparison between groups should be as equitable as possible, meaning that subjects in each group should have an equal chance of receiving or being exposed to the interventions.

Ideally, this comparability is achieved through randomization, where interventions are randomly allocated to the groups. Effective randomization results in groups that are nearly identical in their characteristics at the outset (baseline). This comparability must be maintained throughout the study. Participants in each group should remain similar and comparable, except for their exposure to the interventions. They should receive the same cointerventions, undergo identical assessments, have outcomes measured in the same manner, and avoid dropping out of the study for reasons unrelated to the intervention exposure.

Any factor that undermines the maintenance of such comparability and introduces systematic differences between study groups, an be a potential source of bias.

The main biases that can occur in an interventional study can be categorized as follows, according to the different phases when they can occur:

1. Selection bias: bias that occurs when the sample population is not representative of the target population or when study groups are systematically different from each other.
2. Performance bias: bias due to deviations from the intended interventions.
3. Measurement (or detection) bias: bias in the measurement of the outcome.
4. Attrition bias: bias due to missing outcome information.
5. Reporting bias: bias in the selection of reported results.

11.1.1 Selection Bias

Selection bias results in a sample population that is not representative of the target population (population of interest) or leads to study groups that are systematically different from each other.

In a randomized controlled trial, selection bias can arise when the allocation of participants to treatment and comparison groups is not random, resulting in systematic differences between the groups that could influence study findings (this variant of selection bias is also referred to as allocation bias). To prevent this, researchers should employ robust randomization techniques to ensure unbiased allocation of participants.

Volunteer bias (also known as "response bias") is a type of selection bias that occurs when participants who volunteer for a study have different characteristics compared to the general population of interest. This bias can affect results by reflecting the unique characteristics of the volunteer group, such as higher education levels, higher social status, better health, and greater adherence to treatment. This can limit the generalizability of the findings. Its counterpart is nonresponse bias, which occurs when subjects who do not participate in a study or respond to a survey differ systematically from the rest of the population. Both response and nonresponse biases commonly affect surveys, potentially compromising their validity.

11.1.2 Performance Bias

Performance bias occurs when there are systematic differences between groups in the care that is provided or in exposure to factors other than the interventions of interest. It can arise when patients receive multiple treatments, in addition to the intervention being studied, which could impact the outcome of interest (also called cointervention bias). When there is an imbalance in cointerventions between groups, it is difficult to isolate the effect of the intervention under study from that of cointerventions.

Performance bias can be prevented or mitigated through the blinding (or masking) of study participants and personnel. This ensures that groups receive a similar amount of treatment, including cointerventions. It also reduces the placebo effect by preventing participants and researchers from knowing which intervention was administered, thereby isolating the impact of the primary intervention on the outcome.

11.1.3 Measurement (or Detection) Bias

Measurement (or detection) bias refers to any systematic error occurring during data collection or a systematic difference in how outcomes are detected or measured across study groups. This bias, which can occur if assignment is known, can result in either an overestimate or an underestimate of the treatment or intervention effect. Detection bias can be minimized by using standardized methods to measure outcomes across all groups and by blinding outcome assessors to the treatment group assignments.

11.1.4 Attrition Bias

Attrition bias is a type of selection bias observed in clinical trials of interventions. It occurs when participants drop out of a study, resulting in incomplete outcome data and potentially introducing systematic differences between the groups that could impact study findings.

Attrition can be classified into two types: random and systematic. Random attrition occurs when participants who drop out are similar to those who remain in terms of relevant characteristics. It is considered a random error and does not systematically skew the results. In contrast, systematic attrition involves the selective dropout of participants who differ systematically from those who continue in the study. This type of attrition can introduce bias by creating differences between the study groups that could impact the study's outcomes.

11.1.5 Reporting Bias

Reporting bias occurs when the results of a study are skewed due to how they are reported, leading to systematic differences between reported and unreported findings. This bias can occur when researchers selectively choose to report only certain data while omitting others that might influence their conclusions.

Publication bias occurs when studies with positive results are more likely to be published than those with negative results. This can lead to an overestimation of the effect of a treatment or intervention. Citation bias occurs when researchers selectively cite studies that support their hypothesis or findings while ignoring studies that contradict them. Language or location bias occurs when studies published in languages other than English or, respectively, conducted in certain regions or countries are not included in systematic reviews or meta-analyses, leading to a potential loss of important data. Location bias occurs when studies conducted in certain regions or countries are not included in systematic reviews or meta-analyses, leading to a potential loss of important data.

Reporting bias can be minimized by ensuring that all studies, regardless of their results, are published and made publicly available. Furthermore, study protocols should be registered to ensure that all prespecified outcomes are reported in the final reports. In addition, systematic reviews and meta-analyses should include studies published in all languages and conducted in all regions. Researchers should also be encouraged to publish all their findings, regardless of whether they support their hypothesis or not.

11.2   Hawthorne Effect

The Hawthorne effect occurs when participants in a study change their behavior or outcomes due to awareness of being observed rather than because of the actual intervention being studied, potentially undermining the validity of research findings.

Named after experiments conducted at the Hawthorne Works factory in the 1920s, this effect was initially observed when changes in working conditions, such as lighting, seemed to increase worker productivity. However, productivity changes were later found to correlate more with the increased attention from supervisors during the experiments rather than the specific changes in conditions.

To mitigate the Hawthorne effect, researchers should employ strategies such as randomization to ensure unbiased participant allocation and adopt double-blind procedures whenever possible.

In medical research and other fields, like organizational psychology and education, the Hawthorne effect can pose significant challenges. For instance, consider a study where participants are asked to follow a specific diet or participate in physiotherapy sessions to improve their health. If these participants are aware that they are part of a study and are being closely monitored, they may be motivated to adhere more strictly to the diet or exert more effort in the physiotherapy sessions than they would under normal circumstances. This improvement in behavior may be due not only to the effects of the diet or physiotherapy but also to the positive effect of attention and observation itself on their behavior.

11.3   Biases That Can Occur in Diagnostic Studies

The aim of diagnostic studies is to evaluate the accuracy of a test in diagnosing a specific condition, determining its ability to correctly classify subjects based on the presence or absence of the condition of interest. Diagnostic accuracy studies assess whether a new test can effectively rule in (confirm) or rule out (exclude) a disease. To achieve this, researchers administer both an index test (the new test) and a reference standard test (typically the most reliable existing test, often termed the "gold standard") to all study participants. The results of these tests are then compared to calculate diagnostic parameters such as sensitivity and specificity.

Ideally, diagnostic accuracy studies should enroll consecutive patients (or a random sample of patients) who are at risk for the target condition. Moreover, the participants should represent the full spectrum of patients at risk for the condition. Researchers apply both the index test and the gold standard to all participants, and they compare the results independently and in a blinded manner. Bias can arise in any phase of the study (participant selection, interpretation of test results, ascertainment and confirmation of disease status), potentially leading to inaccurate findings.

11.3.1 Referral Bias

Referral bias occurs when subjects are selected based on the results of a gold standard test, either positive or negative. Because only patients who have undergone the gold standard test are included, participants are chosen systematically and nonrandomly (which is a form of selection bias). As a result, the sample population does not accurately represent the target population, thereby reducing the accuracy and generalizability of study results.

11.3.2 Spectrum Bias

Diseases are usually not all-or-nothing conditions. In medicine, as in biology, there is a range of grey shades between black and white. In medicine and biology, symptoms span a continuum from minimal to severe and from nonspecific to pathognomonic. Ideally, diagnostic studies should capture this full spectrum of disease observed in clinical practice. Therefore, evaluating diagnostic accuracy should encompass patients with clear-cut diagnoses as well as those with ambiguous or uncertain symptoms.

Spectrum bias occurs when the spectrum of disease in subjects included in diagnostic studies differs significantly from that encountered in real-world clinical settings. This bias can be introduced through case-control designs that selectively enroll cases already diagnosed with the condition of interest and controls known to be free of it, thus bypassing diagnostic uncertainties and the nuances of clinical presentation.

Additionally, spectrum bias may arise from nonconsecutive convenience sampling, where patients for whom the index test is challenging are excluded. This selective exclusion can artificially inflate the sensitivity and specificity of the index test, depending on the disease status of excluded patients.

11.3.3 Interpretation and Review Bias

Errors in the interpretation of index test results can significantly impact the validity of diagnostic studies. Excluding patients with unclear or indeterminate test results, such as borderline findings or technically challenging evaluations, may introduce spectrum bias. This exclusion could artificially inflate sensitivity by removing subjects with mild disease who have unclear results. Conversely, it might falsely increase specificity if excluded participants with indeterminate results do not have the target condition. To mitigate this bias, researchers should clearly define in the study protocol how to classify unclear or indeterminate results (i.e., whether to consider them positive or negative).

Review bias can also affect diagnostic test accuracy studies. Diagnostic review bias occurs when the interpreter of the index test results knows the results of the reference standard test. Conversely, index review bias occurs when the interpreter of the reference standard results knows the index test results. Both types of bias can distort study findings by influencing how test results are interpreted.

To minimize these biases, it is crucial to interpret index test results without knowledge of the reference standard results. Similarly, interpreters of the reference standard test should assess results independently of the index test outcomes. Furthermore, reviewers should undergo proper training and possess expertise relevant to the specific diagnostic tests being evaluated. These measures help ensure that diagnostic study results accurately reflect the true performance of the test under investigation.

11.3.4 Differential Verification Bias

Accurate and consistent confirmation of disease is critical in diagnostic accuracy studies. Using two different reference standard tests can introduce variability in the accuracy of disease confirmation, potentially affecting the reliability of the study results.

Verification bias is a type of measurement bias in diagnostic accuracy studies where there is a discrepancy in how disease verification is conducted among different groups of individuals. There are two main types of verification bias: partial verification bias and differential verification bias.

Partial verification bias arises when only some patients undergo the reference standard test, while others do not receive any reference standard test at all. This selective approach can lead to biased estimates of test accuracy.

Differential verification bias occurs when different reference standard tests are applied based on the results of the index test. For instance, an invasive (e.g., angiography, biopsy, and surgery) or expensive reference standard test may be performed only if the index test yields a positive result, potentially inflating sensitivity and specificity estimates.

These biases can distort the true accuracy of the index test and must be carefully considered and minimized in study design and analysis to ensure robust and reliable findings.

11.3.5 Incorporation Bias

Incorporation bias is a form of verification bias that occurs when the outcomes of the index test are included in the reference standard test. This integration can cause an overestimation of the diagnostic accuracy of the index test, as the results of the index test are used to validate the diagnosis. Incorporation bias is especially likely when the reference standard test combines outcomes from multiple tests, including the index test itself. To mitigate incorporation bias, it is essential to maintain the independence of the reference standard test from the index test.

I'm Never Wrong! Logical Fallacies and Cognitive Errors 12

Don't forget that the clinician, in his role as observer, if he wants to see things truly as they are, must start with a clean slate, devoid of any preconceptions regardless of their origins. Magendie reportedly said that in the laboratory he had to experiment like an animal. I would almost say that the clinical observer must adhere to this precept, at least in the first operation, which must lead him to the observation of pathological facts. The harvest being done, he can then reason as much as he wants, relying on freely stated facts. But first he must, as much as possible, free himself from all preoccupation, from all prejudice, to have, in a word, all his freedom of mind.

—Jean-Martin Charcot, *Leçons du Mardi à la Salpêtrière*, April 10, 1888

The patient: Doctor X told me that I was suffering from paralysis agitans; another told me it might be Huntington's disease.

Mr. Charcot: Alas! Alas! Alas! And four times Alas!

—Jean-Martin Charcot, *Leçons du Mardi à la Salpêtrière*, July 3, 1888

In the complex realm of clinical decision-making, physicians face subtle influences that can shape their judgments. Logical fallacies and cognitive errors are common

F. Brigo, *Charcot's Lesson*, Neurocultural Health and Wellbeing, https://doi.org/10.1007/978-3-031-71221-0_12

in medicine, often leading to incorrect diagnoses and treatments, and potentially resulting in adverse patient outcomes.

Recognizing that everyone is susceptible to errors fosters greater tolerance and respect when assessing colleagues' mistakes, as highlighted by Charcot's lament "alas!". Acknowledging our fallibility emphasizes the importance of adopting strategies to minimize errors and identifying common pitfalls to avoid repetition. While errors are human, persisting in them is detrimental.

Awareness of these pitfalls and their potential impact is crucial for mitigating their influence on clinical decision-making, representing a universal strategy applicable to all cognitive biases and logical fallacies. Implementing specific strategies tailored to navigate these biases effectively can enhance diagnostic precision and optimize patient outcomes.

Below, I provide a list and brief overview of common cognitive biases encountered in clinical practice. This compilation, though not exhaustive, highlights 31 significant biases that frequently affect everyday clinical practice. Thirty-one cognitive biases, one for each day of the month: Understanding one bias a day keeps errors at bay! Awareness and understanding of these biases can serve as a daily reminder to reduce errors and improve clinical judgment.

12.1   Cognitive Biases

12.1.1 Affective Error

The affective error influences decision-making by unconsciously relying on emotions, feelings, or personal preferences rather than facts and logic. This can lead to various consequences. For example, physicians might avoid conducting a thorough evaluation for a patient they dislike, such as downplaying the significance of dyspnea in a verbally abusive patient. Moreover, recent or emotionally charged experiences can distort judgment, causing clinicians to overestimate the likelihood of a diagnosis because of vivid memories of dramatic cases or legal complications (also known as recency and intensity bias). Affective errors can significantly impact diagnostic accuracy, treatment decisions, and patient outcomes by promoting inappropriate testing—either excessive or insufficient—and hindering accurate diagnoses.

12.1.2 Aggregate Bias and Ecological Fallacy

In medical research and epidemiology, understanding aggregate bias and the ecological fallacy is crucial. These concepts illuminate the complexities of interpreting group-level data and their implications for individual-level conclusions.

Aggregate bias (ecological bias) occurs when conclusions about individual behavior or risk factors are drawn solely from group-level data. For example, studying the relationship between air pollution levels and respiratory diseases across cities can lead to aggregate bias if we assume uniform risks for all individuals within those cities, masking individual variations due to genetics, lifestyle, or other factors.

Ecological fallacy arises when individual-level associations are inferred from group-level data, assuming that population-level patterns apply uniformly to individuals. For instance, correlating a country's chocolate consumption with its Nobel Prize winners might lead to the fallacy of assuming that chocolate improves individual intellect uniformly, neglecting confounding factors and individual differences.

To mitigate these errors, researchers should prioritize collecting individual-level data whenever feasible, recognizing that group-level patterns may not reflect individual realities. Ecological associations provide hypotheses but require validation at the individual level. In clinical practice, personalized treatment approaches should be favored over assumptions that what benefits a group will benefit every patient. Embracing precision medicine, which tailors treatments based on individual characteristics, ensures that care is more targeted and effective.

In reporting aggregate data, researchers should clarify that findings apply to populations rather than universally to individuals, emphasizing the need for personalized interpretation and application in clinical decision-making.

12.1.3 Ambiguity Effect

The ambiguity effect is a cognitive bias where people tend to avoid options with unknown probabilities and prefer those with known probabilities, even if less favorable. In medicine, ambiguity can arise when there's uncertainty about diagnosis or treatment. This bias may lead physicians to choose a treatment known to have a probability of success, even if less effective than options with uncertain outcomes, potentially leading to suboptimal patient care.

To mitigate this bias, it is important to encourage physicians to consider all treatment options, including those with unknown probabilities. This approach aims to ensure that the patient receives the most effective care possible.

12.1.4 Anchoring

Anchoring bias is a cognitive bias in medicine where physicians rely heavily on initial information (the "anchor") when making subsequent judgments or diagnoses. For example, if a physician initially suspects osteoporosis as the cause of a patient's back pain, they may overlook other possible causes even when evidence suggests otherwise. This initial impression becomes a mental reference point, influencing further assessments during history taking, physical examination, and test interpretation across various medical fields.

This bias can lead to diagnostic overshadowing, where subsequent symptoms or findings are interpreted through the lens of the initial diagnosis. For instance, if a patient with a heart condition complains of fatigue, the physician might attribute all symptoms to the heart issue, potentially missing other underlying problems. Anchoring bias often interacts with confirmation bias, where physicians selectively seek evidence that supports their initial hypothesis while disregarding contradictory information.

To mitigate anchoring bias, physicians should be aware of this tendency and actively challenge their initial impressions. They should systematically consider and generate a list of alternative diagnoses, avoiding premature closure on a single explanation. Actively seeking information that challenges the initial anchor and remaining open to revising hypotheses based on new data is crucial. Discussing cases with colleagues can provide fresh perspectives and help avoid tunnel vision. Effective communication with patients is also essential to explain the diagnostic process, acknowledge uncertainty, and encourage patients to share additional symptoms.

12.1.5 Ascertainment Bias

In medical research, ascertainment bias occurs when clinical judgment is distorted by preconceived expectations, leading to observations that align with those expectations. This pervasive error encompasses various biases and is commonly encountered in clinical trials, where knowledge of participants' interventions can influence results. Ascertainment bias may be introduced by those administering or receiving the intervention, investigators assessing outcomes, or report writers describing trial results. Implementing blinding procedures for participants and researchers can mitigate the impact of ascertainment bias on study outcomes.

12.1.6 Authority Bias and the Bandwagon Effect

Authority bias is a cognitive bias where opinions and instructions from authority figures are unquestioningly accepted and followed. This bias is pervasive in the doctor-patient relationship, medical teams, and training programs. Clinicians of higher status often dictate healthcare decisions, prioritizing symptoms and ordering investigations based on their experience.

Addressing and mitigating authority bias is crucial within healthcare structures as blindly trusting experts can lead to errors. It is important to recognize that even experienced clinicians are susceptible to cognitive biases. Friendship bias, a variant of authority bias, occurs when decisions are influenced by colleagues who are also friends.

The bandwagon effect, closely related to authority bias, describes how people are more likely to adopt trends or beliefs if others do the same. In medicine, this manifests when clinicians adopt popular treatments despite limited evidence. For instance, steroids for acute spinal cord injuries became a standard, based on initial studies in the 1990s, despite later scrutiny questioning their benefits.

The bandwagon effect can lead to the widespread adoption of treatments that may not be effective or could be harmful, highlighting the need for the critical appraisal of medical practices based on robust evidence.

12.1.7 Availability Bias

Availability bias is a cognitive bias that significantly impacts medical decision-making by causing clinicians to rely on readily accessible information or memorable cases rather than considering a broader range of evidence. Common diagnoses and recent, emotionally impactful cases are more easily recalled (recent case bias), while unusual or dramatic cases also stand out and influence decision-making (significant case bias).

For instance, an emergency physician assessing a patient with chest pain may be unduly influenced by a recent encounter with a rare cardiac condition, potentially overshadowing other possible diagnoses.

Availability bias can lead to the neglect of less frequent yet important diagnoses, resulting in potential misdiagnoses and the preference for treatments based on past successes rather than evidence. To counteract availability bias, clinicians should actively consider a spectrum of diagnoses, encompassing both common and rare conditions.

12.1.8 Base-Rate Neglect

Base-rate neglect refers to a cognitive bias where individuals disregard the true prevalence (base rate) of a disease or condition when making decisions. Base rates indicate how likely an event is in a specific population. In medical contexts, understanding base rates is crucial because overlooking them can lead to diagnostic errors. For example, clinicians might focus excessively on rare conditions or underestimate common ones. This can result in both overdiagnosis and underdiagnosis, along with inappropriate treatments.

For instance, if a physician assumes that a patient has a rare disease based on a single symptom without considering its prevalence in the general population, unnecessary tests or treatments may be prescribed. Physicians are particularly prone to base-rate neglect when encountering rare conditions, increasing the likelihood of diagnostic errors.

To counteract base-rate neglect, physicians should be mindful of the prevalence of conditions within the broader population when making clinical decisions. This awareness helps ensure more accurate diagnoses and appropriate management plans.

12.1.9 Belief Bias

Belief bias is a cognitive bias that significantly influences medical decision-making by causing individuals to assess the validity of arguments based on how well they align with existing beliefs rather than on an objective evaluation of evidence. This bias can affect clinical reasoning, diagnostic accuracy, and treatment decisions in medical practice.

In clinical settings, clinicians may dismiss research findings that contradict their beliefs or favor diagnoses that align with their preconceptions, potentially leading to misdiagnoses. Similarly, patients might reject evidence-based treatments that conflict with their personal beliefs.

To mitigate belief bias, clinicians should receive regular training in evidence-based medicine and strive to evaluate evidence objectively, independent of their initial beliefs. This approach helps ensure more accurate diagnoses and appropriate treatment decisions based on the best available evidence.

12.1.10 Blind Spot Bias

Blind spot bias refers to the common belief among physicians that they are less susceptible to biases than others. This belief arises from their confidence in their own introspection and clinical expertise, which can lead to overconfidence in their decision-making abilities. As a result, physicians may fail to recognize how cognitive biases can influence their diagnostic reasoning.

This bias often develops over years of experience and expertise. Seasoned physicians refine their diagnostic skills and develop well-established illness scripts. However, this familiarity with patterns and conditions may cause them to overlook their own biases, assuming their judgment is always clear and objective.

Blind spot bias can contribute to diagnostic errors by causing physicians to dismiss alternative hypotheses too quickly or overlook rare conditions. It also fosters overconfidence, leading clinicians to rely excessively on intuition while disregarding conflicting evidence. This overconfidence can result in missed diagnoses or inappropriate treatments.

Recognizing and addressing blind spot bias is crucial for improving diagnostic accuracy. Physicians should regularly reflect on their decision-making processes, remain open to alternative explanations, and seek feedback to mitigate the impact of this bias on patient care.

12.1.11 Commission Bias

In the complex realm of clinical decision-making, physicians confront the delicate balance between active intervention (commission) and refraining from action (omission), both of which significantly influence patient outcomes.

Commission bias is a cognitive bias where physicians tend to take action, even if unnecessary, rather than choose to do nothing. This bias stems from the ethical principle of beneficence—acting in the patient's best interest.

Consider a physician evaluating a patient with vague symptoms. The inclination to order additional tests, prescribe medications, or perform procedures arises from a proactive approach to prevent potential harm. Commission bias is often more pronounced in overconfident physicians who believe that intervening is always preferable to cautious observation. Despite good intentions, commission bias can result in overdiagnosis, unnecessary treatments, and potential harm. For instance, a physician might order tests or medications that are not clinically warranted, relying on the precautionary principle of "better safe than sorry." To mitigate commission bias, physicians should carefully weigh the risks and benefits of any proposed intervention, proceeding only when the benefits clearly outweigh the potential risks.

Conversely, the opposite bias is known as omission bias (see below).

12.1.12 Confirmation Bias

Confirmation bias involves selectively gathering and interpreting evidence to support existing beliefs while disregarding evidence that contradicts those beliefs. Once a diagnosis is established, there is a tendency to seek out information that confirms it, often overlooking clues that might suggest an alternative diagnosis.

Consider a physician who, after making an initial diagnosis, dismisses any hints from laboratory or radiological results that might suggest a different condition. This bias leads clinicians to perceive what they expect to see.

Confirmation bias plays a crucial role early in the diagnostic process and can reinforce erroneous diagnoses. Subsequent clinicians may accept these initial diagnoses without critically reassessing them—a phenomenon known as diagnostic momentum.

12.1.13 Diagnostic Momentum

In the intricate process of clinical reasoning, physicians often find themselves entangled in the web of diagnostic momentum. This cognitive bias acts like a persistent adhesive, sticking to patients once a diagnosis has been made.

Diagnostic momentum describes the tendency for a diagnostic label to persist once it has been assigned to a patient. It influences subsequent assessments, treatments, and our interpretation of symptoms. For example, if a patient is initially diagnosed with a benign condition like "muscle strain," subsequent healthcare providers may hesitate to reconsider the diagnosis, assuming it is still accurate despite evolving symptoms.

Similar to stubborn adhesive, diagnostic momentum is resistant to removal. It clouds our judgment, making it difficult to see the patient's condition with a fresh perspective. Once a diagnosis is established, it gains authority, shaping how we interpret new information that aligns with the initial label. Colleagues, nurses, and even patients themselves contribute to this momentum by expecting symptoms to fit the diagnosed condition, perpetuating the cycle. Moreover, our minds resist change; adjusting a diagnosis requires significant mental effort, and inertia often leads to continued reliance on the initial assessment.

Diagnostic momentum carries several risks. Clinging to an incorrect diagnosis can lead to overlooking alternative explanations, delaying the recognition of serious conditions, and potentially harming patients. It also narrows the focus of treatment as physicians may continue prescribing therapies that align with the initial diagnosis even if they no longer suit the evolving clinical situation.

12.1.14 Feedback Sanction

In the complex realm of healthcare, clinicians continually make decisions that directly impact patient outcomes. However, the crucial feedback loop, essential for learning and improvement, often remains incomplete. Feedback sanction refers to the absence of timely, honest feedback, which hampers clinicians' ability to recognize and correct their errors. This lack of feedback can lead to the unawareness of mistakes and a failure to take necessary corrective actions.

Feedback sanction can create ignorance traps and time-delay biases, where errors may go unnoticed or have delayed consequences. This perpetuates blind spots in clinical practice, potentially compromising patient safety. Establishing a culture of open communication and feedback among healthcare professionals is essential to mitigate feedback sanction. This culture promotes the identification and prompt resolution of diagnostic errors, ensuring continuous learning and improvement in patient care.

12.1.15 Framing Effect

The framing effect is a cognitive bias that influences how physicians respond to different choices based on how they are presented. For instance, when presented with a treatment option framed in positive terms, physicians may be more inclined to choose it, even in the absence of robust evidence supporting its efficacy. The way information is framed can significantly impact decision-making.

For example, presenting a treatment's success rate as "80% survival" might sway clinicians toward choosing that treatment, whereas framing the same data as "20% mortality" could lead to a different decision.

The framing effect also extends to risk communication. Different presentations may emphasize benefits (e.g., "This drug reduces heart attack risk by 30%") or highlight risks (e.g., "Without this drug, you have a 30% chance of a heart attack"). Such framing influences treatment decisions; positive framing may lead to over-treatment, while negative framing could result in undertreatment. Patients' perceptions of risk are also shaped by how information is framed.

Clinicians should be cautious about how they present information, ensuring to provide a balanced view that includes both positive and negative aspects of treatment options. Involving patients in discussions about framing and understanding their preferences and values are essential steps in shared decision-making.

12.1.16 Fundamental Attribution Error

Fundamental attribution error occurs when physicians place undue emphasis on dispositional or personality factors and neglect situational and environmental factors when explaining social behavior. This psychological bias stems from a tendency to focus on the individual (the actor) rather than considering broader contextual influences. Additionally, clinicians often observe patients' behaviors more readily than the intricate network of external factors shaping those behaviors.

An example of this error is when a physician assumes that a patient is noncompliant with their medication regimen due to laziness or forgetfulness, without fully considering other potential factors, such as medication cost or access to transportation.

To mitigate fundamental attribution errors, clinicians should actively explore alternative explanations for a patient's behavior, even if the initial explanation seems plausible. It is crucial to resist the temptation of simplistic attributions by thoroughly evaluating the patient's context, including social determinants of health and life circumstances. Moreover, cultivating a strong patient-provider relationship, fostering empathy, and demonstrating understanding are essential to effectively uncover situational nuances.

12.1.17 Gambler's Fallacy

In the intricate world of clinical decision-making, healthcare professionals often encounter patterns and probabilities. The gambler's fallacy, a cognitive bias rooted in misperceptions of probability, can significantly impact medical judgments.

This error can be illustrated with a coin-flip example. If a coin lands heads up multiple times in a row, people tend to believe that tails is "due" to balance the sequence. However, this belief is false because the gambler's fallacy ignores the independence of random events: each coin flip or clinical encounter is unrelated to previous ones.

The gambler's fallacy occurs when individuals mistakenly believe that chance events are self-correcting. Specifically, they assume that if a certain outcome has occurred frequently, the opposite outcome is more likely to happen next. For instance, a physician assessing a patient with recurrent migraines may erroneously believe that because the patient has experienced multiple episodes recently, the next episode is less likely to occur soon.

In medicine, assuming that a patient's future outcomes are influenced by past events can lead to diagnostic errors or inappropriate treatment decisions. To mitigate this error, physicians should recognize that each clinical encounter is independent. They should avoid the trap of expecting self-correction where none exists.

12.1.18 Hindsight Bias

In the intricate landscape of clinical practice, healthcare professionals constantly evaluate decisions made in retrospect. The hindsight bias, also known as the "I-knew-it-all-along" phenomenon, significantly influences how we perceive past events. It refers to our tendency to see past events as more predictable than they actually were. After an outcome occurs, we often believe we "knew it all along," even if the situation was uncertain at the time.

For example, imagine a physician reviewing a patient's case after making a rare diagnosis. The physician may erroneously assume that the diagnosis was obvious, neglecting the initial uncertainty.

Hindsight bias distorts our memory of events, as we reconstruct the past to fit the outcome, forgetting the diagnostic challenges we faced and overestimating our own foresight. One risk of hindsight bias is that it affects how we learn from mistakes: if we believe an error was entirely predictable, we may not critically analyze our decision-making process. Thus, it hinders the development of robust clinical reasoning skills.

Recognizing hindsight bias is crucial for quality improvement initiatives. Clinicians should engage in reflective practice, acknowledging the uncertainty they face during decision-making. To mitigate this bias, they should document their thought processes during patient encounters, describing the differential diagnoses considered, even if they seem obvious in hindsight.

12.1.19 Information Bias

Information bias, also known as measurement bias or misclassification, can significantly impact study results and clinical decisions. It occurs when key study variables are incorrectly measured or classified, stemming from systematic differences in how data is obtained from various study groups. This bias can arise from responses to self-administered questionnaires, interview questions, physical measurements, or information in medical records, affecting both observational studies and experiments. It can lead to distorted conclusions and incorrect inferences about the relationship between variables. For example, if a study investigating the effectiveness of a new medication uses different methods to assess outcomes in each group, it could introduce information bias.

Factors contributing to information bias include the lack of blinding (where researchers know group assignments), errors in recording an individual's history, different disease definitions, or varying diagnostic criteria among experts. Additionally, incorrectly calibrated instruments for objective measurements (e.g., weight) or data entry errors can play a significant role.

Information bias can result in the misclassification of disease status, impacting diagnostic accuracy and potentially leading clinicians to base treatment choices on inaccurate data.

Strategies for minimizing information bias in clinical studies include using uniform definitions and criteria across study groups, calibrating measurement instruments properly, and implementing double-blind study designs whenever feasible.

12.1.20 Occam's Error

Occam's error arises from applying the principle of Occam's razor (often referred to as "diagnostic parsimony"), which suggests that when a patient presents with multiple symptoms, clinicians should seek a single diagnosis rather than multiple unrelated ones (see Chap. 8). Occam's error occurs when the physician mistakenly concludes that all symptoms can be explained by a single diagnosis, thereby overlooking the possibility of multiple, concurrent diagnoses. However, if a patient indeed has more than one disease, it remains reasonable to consider several diseases as explanations for their symptoms (while still adhering to the principle of parsimony).

Occam's error is related to anchoring bias (see above).

12.1.21 Omission Bias

Unlike commission bias (see above), omission bias favors inaction over action. It arises from the fear of causing harm through intervention. Imagine a clinician managing a low-risk patient. The reluctance to order tests or initiate treatments stems from the dread of adverse effects or false alarms.

Omission bias often originates from the fear of regret. Physicians may hesitate to act, fearing that an adverse outcome resulting from their intervention would haunt them more than an omission. By erring on the side of caution, omission bias risks underdiagnosing serious conditions. Delayed interventions can have dire consequences.

To mitigate omission bias, clinicians should carefully consider the potential consequences of not taking action and balance this against the risks of intervening unnecessarily. It is crucial to engage patients in informed discussions, explaining the pros and cons of action versus inaction and respecting their autonomy in decision-making. Ultimately, medicine involves managing uncertainty, recognizing that sometimes cautious observation is appropriate while at other times prompt intervention is necessary.

12.1.22 Order Effects

In medical research and clinical practice, the order in which treatments or interventions are administered can significantly influence outcomes. Order effects, also known as sequence effects, refer to differences in participant responses due to the specific order in which they receive treatments. Understanding these effects is crucial for designing robust studies and optimizing patient care.

Participants may improve their performance over time due to practice or familiarity with the task. For instance, repeated cognitive assessments may yield better results in later trials simply because participants have practiced the test. Conversely, participants may perform worse toward the end of an experiment due to mental or physical fatigue, and lengthy or repetitive tasks can lead to decreased attention and accuracy. In addition, prolonged exposure to the same task can lead to boredom, and bored participants may lose motivation, affecting their performance. Finally, participants' responses may be influenced by prior treatments or conditions. For example, estimating the weight of an object may be biased by the weight of the previously estimated object.

The order in which diagnostic tests are performed can impact results. For instance, fatigue during a long imaging session may affect interpretation accuracy. Treatment sequencing (i.e., administering treatments in a specific order) may also affect patient outcomes.

Researchers can use counterbalancing techniques to minimize order effects. For instance, they can randomize the order of treatments across participants to distribute potential biases evenly, introduce breaks between tasks to reduce fatigue and boredom, or allow participants to recover before proceeding to the next intervention.

12.1.23 Patient Satisfaction Error

Patient satisfaction error occurs when healthcare providers prioritize patient satisfaction over medical outcomes. This bias can lead to overprescribing of medications, unnecessary testing, and other interventions that may not be medically necessary. For example, prescribing antibiotics to a patient with flu or another uncomplicated viral infection, despite their clinical ineffectiveness, increases the risk of antibiotic resistance, with negative consequences for public health and individuals.

While patient satisfaction is an important aspect of healthcare, it should not be the sole determinant in medical decision-making. High patient satisfaction scores do not necessarily correlate with better health outcomes. Clinicians should prioritize medical efficacy and safety when making decisions, ensuring interventions are justified based on evidence-based medicine rather than solely to satisfy patient expectations.

Involving patients in shared decision-making is essential. This approach considers patients' perspectives and priorities, providing them with information to make informed choices while aligning treatments with medical necessity and best practices. This balance promotes patient-centered care without compromising medical standards.

12.1.24 Playing the Odds

Clinicians constantly make decisions based on incomplete information. Playing the odds involves assessing probabilities and choosing the most likely diagnosis or treatment strategy. This exercise can be quite subjective and involves diagnostic reasoning, which is the process by which clinicians determine the most probable diagnosis or treatment plan. While not arbitrary, this process can be influenced by cognitive biases.

Diagnostic reasoning entails gathering data from the patient's history and physical examination and constructing a hypothesis about the underlying disease based on the clinician's interpretation of the facts. The strength of the diagnosis will depend on how effectively the clinician collects and integrates information. There may not always be a singular correct approach to applying diagnostic and therapeutic strategies to a specific case.

When seeking explanations, clinicians should remember that common conditions typically present more frequently. While patients can indeed develop rare illnesses, these occurrences are uncommon. Therefore, unusual symptoms and findings are more likely to represent an atypical manifestation of a common problem rather than an entirely rare illness.

12.1.25 Premature Closure

In the fast-paced world of clinical practice, physicians often face time constraints and pressure to make rapid decisions. Premature closure, a cognitive error, occurs when clinicians arrive at a diagnosis or treatment plan too quickly, failing to consider alternative possibilities. This bias can lead to missed diagnoses, delayed interventions, and suboptimal patient care.

Premature closure involves jumping to conclusions without thoroughly exploring all relevant options. It occurs when clinicians stop collecting data prematurely, assuming they have already identified the correct diagnosis or treatment.

For instance, imagine a physician encountering a patient with chest pain. If the physician quickly attributes it to acid reflux without considering other cardiac or pulmonary causes, premature closure may occur.

Clinicians often rely on pattern recognition to expedite decision-making. While this heuristic is valuable, it can lead to premature closure if applied too rigidly. Anchoring bias (fixating on initial information) and availability bias (relying on readily available examples) contribute to premature closure as physicians may latch onto the first plausible explanation without critically evaluating other possibilities.

The danger of premature closure is that it can lead to overlooking less common or atypical conditions. For example, attributing all abdominal pain to gastrointestinal causes may result in missing appendicitis or ovarian torsion. Furthermore, it may lead to inadequate diagnostic testing: clinicians may order unnecessary tests if they prematurely settle on a diagnosis, or conversely, they may fail to order essential tests due to overconfidence.

Strategies for avoiding premature closure include encouraging deliberate thinking and reflection, taking time to consider alternative explanations in a comprehensive differential diagnostic process, and seeking input from colleagues to challenge initial impressions.

12.1.26 Representativeness Restraint

Representativeness restraint is a cognitive bias that can occur in medicine when a clinician hesitates to consider a diagnosis because the patient's presentation does not match the typical pattern. This type of bias can lead to diagnostic errors and inappropriate treatment. For example, if a physician only searches for the classic manifestations of diseases, they may overlook atypical variants.

Representativeness restraint is particularly common among students and more junior staff. If clinicians have learned from textbooks, they may expect that patients will present exactly as described. However, patients often present atypically, and few conform precisely to textbook descriptions. In medicine, it is crucial to recognize when an unusual presentation still fits the profile of an illness.

This bias can result in overlooking less common or atypical conditions. Clinicians may prematurely settle on a diagnosis without fully evaluating the patient's unique features. Therefore, if they focus solely on the typical presentation, they may delay appropriate treatment for less common conditions, such as attributing all chest pain to acid reflux and overlooking acute coronary syndrome.

To mitigate representativeness restraint, clinicians should remain vigilant, actively seeking findings that do not fit the typical pattern, being open to alternative explanations, considering diverse possibilities, and avoiding hasty conclusions. This approach enhances diagnostic accuracy and ensures optimal care for patients.

12.1.27 Search Satisfaction

Nowadays, healthcare professionals frequently and increasingly engage in information-seeking behaviors. Search satisfaction, a cognitive phenomenon, refers to the tendency to stop searching for additional information once a satisfactory answer is found. While this approach can enhance efficiency, it also carries risks.

For example, if a physician diagnoses a patient with a common condition based on a few symptoms, they may fail to consider other, less common conditions that could also be causing the symptoms. In radiology, search satisfaction is referred to as satisfaction of search error. It occurs when the reporting radiologist fails to continue searching for additional abnormalities after identifying an initial one. This premature termination of the search can lead to missed findings, which may be crucial for accurate diagnosis and patient management.

12.1.28 Sunk Cost Fallacy

Healthcare professionals often grapple with resource allocation, treatment choices, and patient management. The sunk cost fallacy, a cognitive bias, significantly influences how clinicians evaluate past investments and make future decisions.

This bias can occur when a clinician continues to invest resources in a treatment or intervention despite evidence that it is not effective, leading to inappropriate treatment decisions. For example, if a physician prescribes a medication that proves ineffective, they may continue to do so because the patient has already invested time and money in the treatment. The sunk cost fallacy is rooted in economic theory but applies broadly to human behavior, including medicine. It suggests that individuals tend to overvalue resources already invested (sunk costs), such as time, money, or emotional involvement, and allow these sunk costs to influence future decisions. Moreover, the greater the effort or resources already invested, the more challenging it becomes to abandon a failing strategy.

The sunk cost fallacy can result in the persistence of ineffective treatments as clinicians may hesitate to change course due to the perceived loss of prior investments. In healthcare systems, this bias can also affect decisions about equipment, facilities, and research projects. However, rational resource allocation should prioritize future benefits over past expenditures.

One effective strategy to counteract the sunk cost fallacy is to evaluate the effectiveness of a treatment based on objective data rather than previous investments alone. This approach encourages clinicians to make decisions based on current evidence and patient outcomes, promoting more effective and patient-centered care.

12.1.29 Sutton's Slip

Physicians often face the challenge of efficiently arriving at accurate diagnoses and treatment plans. Sutton's slip emphasizes the importance of bypassing unnecessary steps and focusing on the most direct path to a solution. In medicine, this principle encourages clinicians to prioritize relevant investigations and interventions while avoiding superfluous tests or procedures.

Sutton's slip is named after Willie Sutton, a notorious bank robber in the early twentieth century. When asked why he robbed banks, Sutton reportedly replied, "Because that's where the money is." This succinct philosophy underscores the importance of targeting the most relevant and effective actions.

In the context of clinical decision-making, clinicians should prioritize investigations or interventions that directly address the patient's chief complaint or most concerning symptoms. They should avoid routine or nonspecific tests that do not significantly contribute to the diagnostic process. When faced with complex presentations, it is important to break down the problem into its essential components and address each systematically rather than pursuing an exhaustive battery of tests.

By bypassing irrelevant steps, Sutton's slip optimizes resource allocation, reducing costs associated with unnecessary tests and procedures.

12.1.30 Triage Cueing

Triage cueing is a cognitive bias that can occur in medicine when a clinician's subsequent thought process about a patient's presentation is influenced by the initial triage assessment. When a patient arrives at an emergency department, they undergo triage—a focused nursing assessment to summarize the problem, estimate urgency, and assign the patient to a specific area. Due to the brief nature of triage assessments, they can be susceptible to various biases, such as anchoring bias, diagnostic momentum, and availability bias, which may persist through subsequent evaluations.

The treating clinician may form initial impressions based on the triage nurse's summary, the assigned triage category, and the geographical location to which the patient is directed. Geographical cues can influence expectations about the severity of patients in different areas. Clinicians might incorrectly assume that patients in lower acuity areas are less seriously ill, potentially overlooking life-threatening conditions.

Further triage cueing errors can arise when a patient is referred to a particular specialty, leading the clinician to evaluate the patient's condition primarily from the perspective of that subspecialty. This can narrow diagnostic considerations and potentially delay appropriate management.

12.1.31 Zebra Retreat

Zebra retreat is a cognitive bias that occurs in medicine when a physician withdraws from considering a rare and unusual diagnosis, despite evidence supporting it, simply because of its rarity. This phenomenon often arises when a rare diagnosis is initially considered in the differential diagnosis but the physician retreats from it due to concerns about being perceived as unrealistic. Factors such as self-consciousness and underconfidence in assuming a very rare diagnosis in a busy emergency department, along with anticipated time and effort required for further investigation, fatigue, distractions, and difficulty accessing relevant subspecialties, can diminish the physician's conviction and lead to the abandonment of the initial hypothesis.

Zebra retreat, also known as the "courage of convictions," is typically associated with base-rate neglect and availability bias. If a physician fails to pursue a rare diagnosis because they cannot recall ever encountering or investigating it before, this may indicate zebra retreat. Conversely, if a physician regularly investigates rare conditions without adequate consideration of their low prevalence, this exemplifies base-rate neglect, potentially leading to unnecessary resource utilization, overdiagnosis, and patient harm.

To mitigate zebra retreat and related biases, clinicians should maintain awareness of both the likelihood of rare diagnoses (base rates) and the availability of evidence when making diagnostic decisions. Balancing thoroughness with efficiency is crucial: while it is important to consider rare conditions when indicated by evidence, an overzealous pursuit of zebras should be avoided when common conditions are more probable.

12.2   How to Get Rid of Cognitive Errors

Eliminating cognitive errors is challenging because many are ingrained in human reasoning and stem from the inherent structure of our thought processes. They often represent extremes of a cognitive spectrum, each with its own rules and validity, which can lead to errors when pushed to their limits.

Below, I provide a decalogue of useful approaches to mitigate these biases and enhance your practice:

1. Awareness and education: stay informed about common cognitive biases and their potential impact. Engage in educational activities that highlight these biases and their implications. Avoid factors that increase error risks, such as stress, high decision density, interruptions, distractions, fatigue, sleep deprivation, and emotional disruptions.
2. Differential diagnosis: maintain a comprehensive list of potential diagnoses for each patient. Routinely and systematically evaluate all relevant possibilities, including both common and rare conditions, even if the initial diagnosis seems probable. Resist the temptation of simplistic conclusions and consider the patient's context, social determinants of health, and life circumstances.
3. Checklists and decision aids: use structured checklists to guide diagnostic reasoning and follow evidence-based treatment algorithms to minimize bias in therapeutic decisions. Gain a deeper understanding of epidemiological features, such as incidence, prevalence, seasonality, and geographic distribution of disorders.
4. Second opinions and peer review: seek second opinions for challenging cases. Regularly discuss cases with colleagues to explore alternative perspectives and challenge assumptions.
5. Embrace uncertainty: acknowledge that medicine involves uncertainty. Rely on empirical data rather than intuition alone. Humility in medicine and in life pays off.
6. Patient-centered approach: involve patients in discussions about risks, benefits, and treatment options. Understand individual patient values and preferences to tailor decisions accordingly.

7. Reflective practice: analyze diagnostic and treatment errors to uncover underlying biases. Continuously evaluate your decision-making process and learn from your own errors.
8. Time management: allocate sufficient time for patient encounters to avoid rushed decisions. Pause to consider alternative explanations and allow time for thoughtful reflection.
9. Evidence-based practice: Base decisions on rigorous research, clinical guidelines, and systematic reviews. Challenge assumptions based on new evidence as it becomes available.
10. Open mindset: be open to revising initial hypotheses based on evolving information. Foster a culture where you and your colleagues can openly discuss errors and explore situational nuances, promoting empathy and understanding.

Further Reading

Howard J. Cognitive errors and diagnostic mistakes. Cham: Springer; 2018.
Morgenstern J. Cognitive errors in medicine: the common errors. First10EM. 15 Sept 2015. https://doi.org/10.51684/FIRS.726.
Raz M, Pouryahya P, editors. Decision making in emergency medicine: biases, errors and solutions. Singapore: Springer; 2021.

Evidence Is Much but Not All: Rethinking Evidence-Based Medicine

13

> *In short, it seems to be a common case, quite ordinary. A substantial number of such cases have been seen at the clinic this year, and we have discussed them extensively. However, perhaps in this specific instance, upon closer examination, we will find something noteworthy to observe.*
>
> —Jean-Martin Charcot, *Leçons du Mardi à la Salpêtrière, June 19, 1888*

At first glance, the concept of Evidence-Based Practice (EBP) might seem self-explanatory. After all, it's right there in the name, right? Well, not quite. The term "evidence-based practice" can be misleading. Some labels are far from neutral; they evoke specific reactions or associations. One might wonder whether the emphasis on "evidence" in EBP's name contributes to why some still view it with suspicion, perceiving it as elitist or exclusive—something confined within the "ivory tower" of academia. For some, evidence is Evidence (with a capital "E"), and Cochrane is its prophet. When most systematic reviews conclude that "robust evidence from randomized controlled trials is lacking and further studies are needed," physicians might feel compelled to comply, reinforcing the notion that evidence reigns supreme.

In reality, however, EBP is much more nuanced. It is a paradigm that integrates scientific research findings into clinical decision-making, allowing healthcare professionals to base their actions on reliable data rather than tradition or intuition.

According to David Sackett (1934–2015), widely considered the "father" of EBP, "Evidence-based medicine is the conscientious, explicit, and judicious use of current best evidence in making decisions about the care of individual patients. The practice of evidence-based medicine means integrating individual clinical expertise with the best available external clinical evidence from systematic research." Above all, EBP is practical and pragmatic, designed for utility rather than abstract

F. Brigo, *Charcot's Lesson*, Neurocultural Health and Wellbeing, https://doi.org/10.1007/978-3-031-71221-0_13

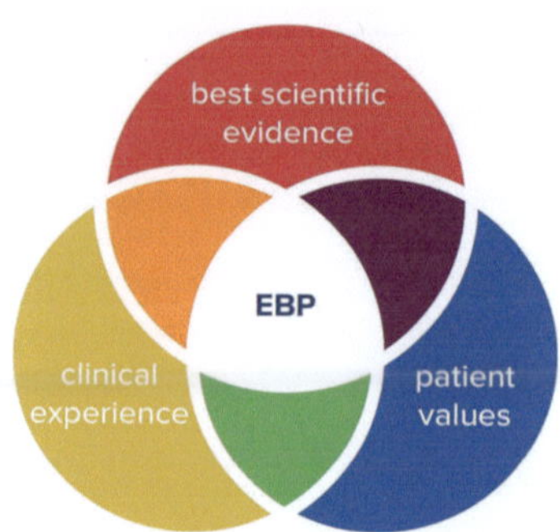

Fig. 13.1 Evidence-based practice (EBP) encompasses three domains: best available evidence, clinical expertise, and patient values. They should be integrated into clinical decision-making, aiming to improve patient outcomes and to enhance the quality of care provided

theorizing. It serves as a tool for guiding clinical decisions by harmonizing three critical elements: clinician expertise, patient values, and the best available evidence. Evidence alone, while essential, is neither sufficient nor all-powerful. EBP thrives from the productive interplay of these three domains, forming a balanced approach to patient care (Fig. 13.1).

The practice of EBP adheres to specific core principles. It is conscientious, explicit, and judicious—grounded in logic and rationality, not mysticism or ideology. Practitioners of EBP are able to clearly articulate the reasons and justifications for their actions. Its methodology emphasizes transparency and reproducibility, ensuring that decisions are based on a clear process rather than intuition or guesswork. EBP is not an abstract art form but a practical, teachable approach, focused on applying the best available evidence—even when that evidence is not definitive.

This commitment to using the best possible evidence demands a rigorous search for and identification of the most current and optimal data. Evidence in EBP is not accepted on blind faith but is scrutinized and critically assessed. As a result, the process of EBP unfolds in stages, systematically working to identify the most relevant information in a timely and efficient manner.

Each day, tens of thousands of new scientific articles flood databases like PubMed or Scopus. Amidst this overwhelming volume of information, EBP provides a structured framework—a "compass and map" to help healthcare professionals find the answers they need. So, don't panic—just stay the course and follow the evidence!

13.1   Step by Step Toward the Goal

The process of Evidence-Based Practice (EBP) consists of several steps, all of which conveniently start with the letter "A"—making them easy to remember:

1. Ask a question
2. Acquire evidence
3. Appraise evidence critically
4. Apply evidence
5. Assess the effectiveness of the entire process

13.1.1 Ask a Question

The first step is to formulate a clinical question that is relevant to the patient's care. The question should be focused and answerable using the best available evidence. Questions can be good or bad. A good question is not one that already has an answer but rather one that could potentially be answered. In other words, a good question is well formulated, enabling the identification of an answer if it exists. A good question is an answerable question.

How do you develop a good clinical question? An effective strategy is to follow the PICO framework, where P stands for the target patient population, I stands for intervention, C stands for comparison or alternative to the intervention of interest, and O stands for outcomes (Table 13.1).

Whenever necessary or appropriate, you can add further details to your PICO question. You can specify details about your population (e.g., elderly, adolescents, pregnant women) and intervention (e.g., method of administration, dose) and also include additional components such as study type (e.g., randomized controlled trial), setting (e.g., outpatients, hospital, emergency department), geographic area (e.g., Africa), specific time frame, etc. These details will influence your search strategy and the results you may obtain. Adding more details can increase result precision but may reduce search sensitivity and the likelihood of finding sufficient articles.

13.1.2 Acquire Evidence

The next step is to search for evidence to answer the clinical question. This involves searching the literature for relevant studies using a search strategy developed based on the clinical question framed according to the PICO format. The search strategy should aim for a balance between sensitivity and specificity to identify all studies relevant to the clinical research question.

Table 13.1 Elements of the PICO framework used to structure clinical questions for research or clinical decision-making

Framework of a good clinical question	
Population	What is the target population?
Intervention	What is the intervention of interest?
Comparator(s)	What is/are the alternative(s) to the intervention?
Outcome(s)	What is/are the outcome(s) of interest?

The PICO framework for a good clinical question involves four key components. P—patient, population, or problem—describes the characteristics of the patient or population under consideration, including relevant demographics and conditions. I—intervention, exposure, or issue—specifies the main intervention, exposure, or issue being studied or managed. C—comparison—identifies any alternative interventions, exposures, or issues being compared to the intervention or issue described in "I" (if applicable). O—outcome—defines the outcomes or effects of interest for the patient or population described in "P" when considering the intervention or issue described in "I"

Searches are typically conducted in electronic databases that list scientific and medical articles. Not all databases are the same; each specializes in certain areas.

One of the most widely used and sought-after medical databases is MEDLINE (accessed through PubMed). Another significant database is Embase. PsycINFO is dedicated to mental health literature, while CINAHL covers biomedicine, healthcare, nursing, and allied health articles. Scopus, Web of Science, and Google Scholar encompass many scientific disciplines, and the Cochrane Library is renowned for systematic reviews.

A valuable evidence-based resource is the Trip medical database, a search engine that helps users find high-quality clinical research evidence (available at www.tripdatabase.com). It allows users to search PICO (population, intervention, comparison, outcome) questions and presents results ordered by methodological quality, date (more recent first), and relevance. The interface is intuitive and user-friendly, categorizing evidence sources with color codes (e.g., primary evidence coded as red, secondary evidence as green).

Another useful tool is the Epistemonikos database (available at http://www.epistemonikos.org), a large repository of healthcare systematic reviews. It integrates with a platform called L·OVE (Living OVerview of Evidence), which contains and maps the best evidence relevant to health decision-making as soon as it becomes available (available at http://app.iloveevidence.com).

Before developing your search strategy, it is important to determine which databases are most appropriate for your research question and to consider potential differences in how search queries are structured and utilized.

13.1.2.1 Develop the Search Terms

Developing a search strategy begins by carefully analyzing the research question and identifying the essential concepts and terms relevant to the inquiry. Next, it is crucial to determine the most appropriate search terms and synonyms for each concept. To ensure adequate sensitivity, your search strategy should always encompass terms related to the P (patient, population, or problem) and the I (intervention of interest). Depending on the desired specificity, you may also incorporate terms related to the O (outcomes) and, if applicable, the C (comparator).

13.1.2.2 Combine the Search Terms

Search terms should be combined using Boolean operators in a search query to produce accurate and relevant results. The three most common Boolean operators are AND, OR, and NOT:

- **AND**: when using the AND operator, both search terms must be present in the search results. For example, searching for "epilepsy AND stroke" will retrieve pages that contain both "epilepsy" and "stroke." This operator is useful when you want to find articles that address both concepts simultaneously, such as in studies on epilepsy and stroke co-occurrence.
- **OR**: the OR operator allows either one or both of the search terms to appear in the search results. For instance, searching for "epilepsy OR stroke" will retrieve

pages that contain either "epilepsy," "stroke," or both terms. OR is particularly helpful when you want to include multiple terms or synonyms for a concept, broadening the scope of your search.
- **NOT**: when using the NOT operator, pages containing the specified search term are excluded from the results. For example, searching for "epilepsy NOT stroke" will retrieve pages that mention "epilepsy" but do not include "stroke." NOT is useful for narrowing down search results when specific aspects of a topic are of interest and you wish to exclude irrelevant content.

Additional ways to refine search queries include:

- *Brackets*: brackets are used to group search terms and specify the order of operations. For example, searching for "asthma AND (child OR adolescent)" ensures that results include "asthma" and either "child" or "adolescent."
- *Truncations*: truncation involves using an asterisk (*) to search for variations of a word. For instance, searching for "child*" will retrieve results containing "child," "children," "childhood," etc. Truncation helps capture different forms of a word but should be used cautiously to avoid retrieving irrelevant results.
- *MeSH terms*: medical subject headings (MeSH) are standardized terms used in databases like MEDLINE to describe biomedical concepts. Adding "[Mesh]" after a term, such as "asthma[Mesh]," ensures the retrieval of articles indexed with that specific MeSH term, improving search accuracy.

These strategies enhance the precision and relevance of search results, aiding in efficient literature review and evidence retrieval in research and clinical practice.

13.1.2.3 Refine the Search Strategy

Your search strategy can be enhanced by applying limits or filters to narrow down search results based on specific criteria. PubMed and other databases typically offer a filter bar on search result pages, which enables users to refine their searches using various parameters.

Here are examples of filters that can help refine your search strategy:

- Article type: this filter allows users to limit search results to specific types of articles, such as clinical trials, case reports, reviews, and more.
- Publication date: this filter enables users to restrict search results to articles published within a specific date range.
- Age: this filter allows users to focus search results on articles that pertain to a specific age group, such as infants, children, adults, or the elderly.
- Language: this filter enables users to limit search results to articles published in a specific language.
- Species: this filter allows users to refine search results to articles focused on a particular species, such as humans, animals, or plants.
- Gender: this filter enables users to restrict search results to articles that focus on a specific gender, such as male or female.

By utilizing these filters judiciously, you can effectively narrow down search results to find articles that are most relevant to your specific research needs and objectives.

13.1.3 Appraise Evidence

Once you have identified the evidence to answer your clinical question, the next step is to critically appraise it to determine its validity and applicability to the patient's care. In doing so, you need to consider the principle of the hierarchy of evidence.

13.1.3.1 The Hierarchy of Evidence

The hierarchy of evidence is a framework that ranks the quality of evidence based on the strength of the study design and the risk of bias. The pyramid is divided into different levels, with the highest level at the top, arranged in order of decreasing strength of evidence (Fig. 13.2).

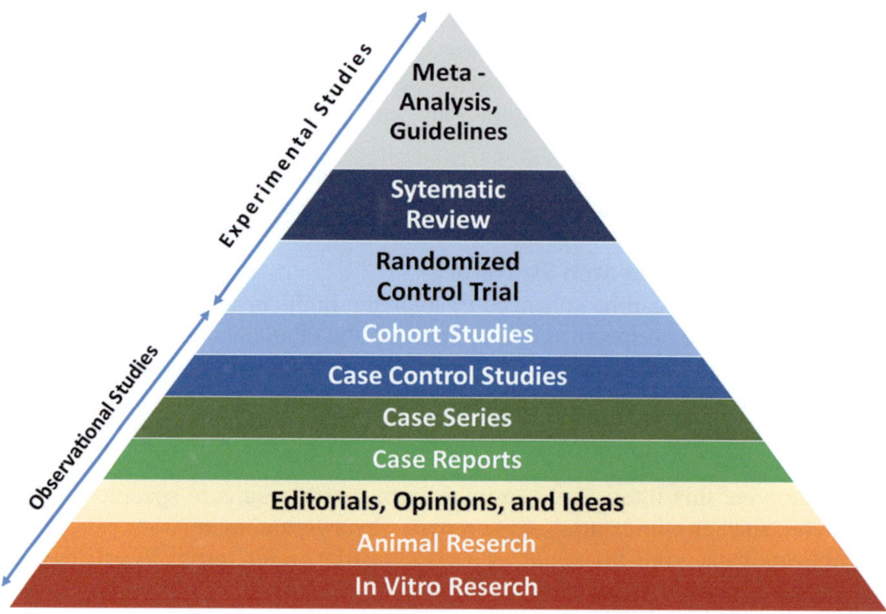

Fig. 13.2 The pyramid of evidence is a hierarchical framework used in evidence-based practice (EBP) to rank different types of research studies based on their methodological rigor and reliability. It helps clinicians and researchers assess the strength of evidence supporting various healthcare interventions or practices. The pyramid typically organizes study designs from lower to higher levels of evidence, with the higher levels generally considered more reliable for informing clinical decisions

At the top of the pyramid, systematic reviews and meta-analyses are considered the highest level of evidence because they provide a comprehensive and unbiased summary of all available evidence on a specific topic. These reviews are based on rigorous methodologies involving systematic literature searches, critical appraisal of study quality, and statistical synthesis of results.

Randomized controlled trials (RCTs) are considered the gold standard for assessing intervention effectiveness. In RCTs, participants are randomly assigned to intervention or control groups to compare outcomes, minimizing bias and confounding variables.

Cohort studies are observational studies that follow a group of individuals over time to determine the incidence of specific outcomes and identify risk factors.

Case-control studies are observational studies that compare individuals with a particular outcome (cases) to those without (controls), useful for investigating rare outcomes and identifying associated risk factors.

Case series are descriptive studies reporting on a group of patients with a specific condition, useful for generating hypotheses and describing clinical features.

Expert opinion represents the lowest level of evidence based on the experience and judgment of individuals or groups of experts. While useful for hypothesis generation and guidance in the absence of other evidence, it lacks the rigor of systematic investigation.

When interpreting or adopting the "pyramid of evidence," several caveats must be considered:

- The hierarchy of evidence is a valid framework under ideal circumstances, assuming each study type within each category is well conducted and free of bias. However, this validity must be proven and cannot be assumed. Randomized controlled trials ideally provide more accurate and reliable evidence than observational studies. However, biased randomized controlled trials can yield lower-quality evidence compared to well-conducted observational studies.
- The hierarchy of evidence encompasses various study designs, all aimed at assessing causal relationships between exposure and outcome. Interventional studies evaluating the impact of interventions (e.g., drugs, surgeries, devices) coexist with studies investigating associations between risk factors and diseases (e.g., hypercholesterolemia and cardiovascular accidents). Certain study designs are more suited to address specific clinical questions. For instance, a case-control study is appropriate for investigating the link between smoking and stroke, whereas a randomized controlled trial is not. Conversely, a placebo-controlled randomized controlled trial is more suitable than a case-control study for evaluating the efficacy of a new migraine medication.

Once you've identified an article that potentially answers your clinical question, the next step is to evaluate the validity of its findings. Begin by focusing on the study's methodology rather than jumping straight to the results. If the methods are robust and reliable, you can then proceed to assess the results. Through this process of seeking and critically appraising evidence, you can identify the most relevant evidence available. Keep in mind that while the highest-quality evidence is ideal, valuable insights can still be drawn from lower-level sources, such as case reports, which contribute to evidence-based practice.

13.1.4 Apply Evidence

The next step involves integrating the best available evidence with clinical expertise and patient values to guide patient care decisions. This includes assessing the benefits and risks of various treatment options while considering the patient's perspective. At this stage, ask yourself if the results will contribute to better patient care. Furthermore, it is crucial to bear in mind that while evidence is significant, it is not the sole factor to consider! Before utilizing the best available evidence to guide your decision-making, evaluate the evidence quality, weigh the balance between benefits and harm, and consider resource utilization. Engaging in meaningful discussions with patients is essential to ensure that treatment choices align with their individual preferences and values, promoting shared decision-making in a patient-centered approach. Striking a balance between evidence-based recommendations and respect for patients' autonomy remains pivotal in every clinical decision.

13.1.5 Assess the Effectiveness of the Entire Process

The final step is to evaluate the effectiveness of the decision and modify the approach as needed. Reflect on how the EBP process influenced your clinical decision, identify any challenges you encountered and how you could overcome them, assess patient and personal satisfaction, reflect on lessons learned, and consider areas for improvement. Especially in the initial stages, searching the literature and critically evaluating evidence can be time-consuming. Don't get discouraged! Like any learning process, mastering EBP requires practice and patience, but the effort pays off. Over time, efficiency and effectiveness will improve. Next time it will definitely be better.

13.2 The Benefits of Evidence-Based Practice

Evidence-based practice has several benefits for patients and healthcare professionals. For patients, EBP ensures they receive the most effective treatments and interventions, thereby strengthening their relationship with healthcare providers. EBP also promotes patient-centered care by involving patients in the decision-making process and considering their values and preferences.

For healthcare professionals, EBP provides a framework for making clinical decisions based on the best available evidence. It promotes lifelong learning and professional development by encouraging healthcare professionals to stay updated with the latest research and evidence. EBP enhances problem-solving strategies and autonomy in clinical decisions and fosters critical and logical reasoning.

Additionally, EBP helps limit wasteful expenditures and optimize resources by protecting against misleading or biased information. It also identifies unresolved issues that warrant further research.

Further Reading

Guyatt G, Rennie D, Meade MO, Cook DJ, editors. Users' guides to the medical literature: a manual for evidence-based clinical practice. 3rd ed. New York: McGraw-Hill; 2015.
Prasad K. Fundamentals of evidence based medicine. New Delhi: Springer; 2013.

How to Critically Appraise a Medical Article

14

> *The well-established existence today of cases of this condition has led to criticism of the definition given by James Parkinson in his remarkable treatise on shaking paralysis (An Essay on the Shaking Palsy, James Parkinson, member of the Royal College of Surgeons, London, 1817). This publication, which has become exceedingly rare today, is a very small work. After much futile searching, I nonetheless possess a copy, which I owe to the great kindness of Dr. Windsor, librarian at the University of Manchester. Despite its brevity, this work contains a wealth of excellent material, and I would strongly encourage one of you to provide a French translation.*
>
> *—Jean-Martin Charcot, Leçons du Mardi à la Salpêtrière, June 12, 1888*

Critical appraisal of a medical article is an essential process for evaluating the reliability, significance, and applicability of clinical research papers. It is a crucial skill for healthcare professionals to ensure they use the best available evidence in clinical practice.

Critical appraisal is a fundamental step in the evidence-based medicine process, aiming to identify the most relevant evidence on a specific topic. By carefully reading and critically evaluating an article, you should determine if it addresses your clinical problem and provides valid results and assess whether these results can be applied to your patient.

Therefore, critical appraisal involves several steps, which can be guided by the following questions in sequential order:

1. Is this article relevant to my clinical question?
2. Are the results valid?

© The Author(s), under exclusive license to Springer Nature Switzerland AG 2024

F. Brigo, *Charcot's Lesson*, Neurocultural Health and Wellbeing, https://doi.org/10.1007/978-3-031-71221-0_14

3. What are the results?

Each question should be answered sequentially with a "yes" or "no," progressing to the next question only if the current one is answered affirmatively. This stepwise approach ensures a thorough evaluation and applies to both treatment and diagnostic articles.

14.1   Is This Article Relevant to My Clinical Question?

The first step is to identify the question that the study aims to answer and to verify if it aligns with your own clinical question. In other words, you need to efficiently and quickly ascertain whether the article in front of you is truly relevant to your needs.

The fundamental premise is clarity about your clinical question. You must clearly understand the type of information you are seeking: the population or type of patients, the problem or disease, the intervention of interest, and the outcome. Formulating your clinical question using the patient/population, intervention, comparison, and outcome (PICO) format helps clarify your objectives.

Scientific articles adhere to a standardized structure. Original articles on therapy or diagnosis typically include the following sections: abstract, introduction, methods, results, discussion (and conclusions), and references. This structured approach facilitates systematic reporting and enables quick information retrieval.

In the article, the clinical question should be explicitly stated in two places: at the beginning of the abstract under the aims/objective section and at the end of the introduction.

Detailed information about the population or patients, and the problem or disease, can be found in the methods section, which should clearly outline inclusion and exclusion criteria. Similarly, details about interventions, diagnostic tests, and outcomes are reported in this section.

Ultimately, it is your responsibility to assess whether and to what extent the article meets your needs. The closer the alignment between the question addressed in the article and your own clinical question, the better. However, some degree of discrepancy may be acceptable. If so, consider that the applicability of the study results to your patients (external validity or generalizability of the study) may not be absolute.

14.2   Are the Results Valid?

The validity of study results should be assessed based on the type of article, whether it pertains to therapy or diagnosis. This consideration takes into account variations in methodology and potential biases specific to each type. When evaluating result validity, attention should primarily (though not exclusively) be focused on the method section to identify biases that could undermine accuracy.

A detailed discussion of systematic errors that may arise in therapy and diagnosis articles is provided in Chap. 11. Understanding the main types of biases is essential for critically appraising study results. While no study is entirely free from bias, minimizing their number and relevance enhances result reliability.

To facilitate methodological evaluation and bias assessment, especially for beginners, using checklists or guiding questions tailored to the type of article (therapeutic or diagnostic) of interest can be particularly helpful.

14.3 What Are the Results?

Once you have determined that the study results are sufficiently valid to warrant further consideration, you can proceed to the next step and assess what the results actually are. This assessment varies depending on the type of study. A therapy article will typically present data on efficacy and tolerability, often including effect size data expressed in various metrics. In contrast, a diagnostic article will focus on the parameters of diagnostic accuracy, such as sensitivity and specificity.

In both cases, it is crucial to evaluate the magnitude of the results and the effect size for each outcome considered (e.g., efficacy, safety, quality of life, sensitivity, specificity). It is important not to conflate statistical significance with clinical relevance. A result may be statistically significant (indicating a real finding) but clinically insignificant. For instance, consider a new painkiller that reduces pain perception by one point on a scale of 0–10 compared to placebo, with a p-value of 0.001. Despite the statistical significance, the clinical relevance of such a small reduction may be questionable.

14.4 Final Remarks

At the conclusion of the critical evaluation of an article, you need to consider how to apply the results to your patients. This step is both the starting point and the culmination of the entire evidence-based process. Once you have reviewed the overall study findings, you must assess whether the study participants are similar enough to the patients in your own practice. Moreover, when deciding how to apply study results, it is essential to integrate the level of evidence with your own clinical experience, the patient's values and preferences, and the balance between potential benefits on one hand and potential harms and costs on the other.

Further Reading

Guyatt G, Rennie D, Meade MO, Cook DJ, editors. Users' guides to the medical literature: a manual for evidence-based clinical practice. 3rd ed. New York: McGraw-Hill; 2015.
Prasad K. Fundamentals of evidence based medicine. New Delhi: Springer; 2013.

Part II

Theory and Practice

Critical Appraisal of a Therapy Article: Randomized Controlled Trial

15

You can use the following checklists to critically appraise an article reporting the results of a randomized controlled trial (RCT). To make this process easier, I have also included a series of notes and tips designed to help you identify methodological flaws more effectively, quickly, and with less effort.

15.1 Is This Article Relevant to My Clinical Question? (Checklist I)

Checklist I: Is This Article Relevant to My Clinical Question?

Are the patients in the study similar enough to those in my clinical question (clinical characteristics, setting)?	No ☐	Yes ☐	Unclear ☐
Is the intervention evaluated in this study the same as that in my clinical question?	No ☐	Yes ☐	Unclear ☐
Is the intervention evaluated in this study available in my clinical practice?	No ☐	Yes ☐	Unclear ☐
Does this article evaluate the outcome/s I am interested in?	No ☐	Yes ☐	Unclear ☐

Supplementary Information The online version contains supplementary material available at https://doi.org/10.1007/978-3-031-71221-0_15.

F. Brigo, *Charcot's Lesson*, Neurocultural Health and Wellbeing, https://doi.org/10.1007/978-3-031-71221-0_15

15.2   Are the Results Valid? Assessment of Accuracy (Internal Validity, Risk of Bias)

15.2.1 Did Participants in the Two Groups Begin with the Same Prognosis? (Selection Bias) (Checklist II)

Checklist II: Did Participants in the Two Groups Begin with the Same Prognosis?

Did participants in the two groups begin with the same prognosis? (Selection bias)			
Has the assignment to treatments been really based on chance alone (random generation)?	No ☐	Yes ☐	Unclear ☐
Was the allocation of patients to treatment predicA in any way (allocation concealment)?	No ☐	Yes ☐	Unclear ☐
At the beginning of the study, were the patients in the two groups similar in demographics, disease severity, or known prognostic factors?	No ☐	Yes ☐	Unclear ☐

15.2.1.1 Notes and Tips

Randomization should truly be a play of chance! In other words, patient assignment must be free from any intentional or unintentional influence that could result in dissimilar groups. Proper randomization methods based purely on chance include coin tosses (an old-fashioned but still valid approach, especially with large participant numbers), drawing numbers from a hat (a simple but effective way to ensure random allocation), using a list of random numbers, or sequentially numbered, sealed, opaque envelopes containing assignment information. In contrast, inadequate methods of randomization, where group allocation can be influenced, include assignments based on days of the week or alternating assignments.

Concealment allocation: chance, not choice! The effectiveness of randomization can be compromised if the investigators are aware of the group assignments before recruiting participants, potentially introducing selection bias. Allocation concealment ensures that those recruiting patients are unaware of the upcoming assignment, maintaining the integrity of randomization. For example, a coin toss or a computer-generated random number list ensures both true randomization and proper allocation concealment. On the other hand, alternating assignments do not guarantee concealment, as the investigator can predict the next group allocation. Remember, allocation must be based on chance, not choice!

Comparability of study groups at baseline: the aim of randomization is to result in groups that are nearly identical at baseline. To evaluate whether randomization has been effective in balancing the features of participants across the study groups, you should examine the table reporting the demographics and clinical features of participants at baseline (usually it is the first table provided in the article). Pay attention to the sample size and the randomization method adopted. The effectiveness of simple randomization (i.e., randomization performed without restriction on allocation) in achieving comparable groups depends on the sample size and the randomization method used. Ideally, tossing a coin is associated with a 50:50 chance of getting a head or a tail. However, with only a few coin tosses, the results may

THE EFFECTIVENESS OF RANDOMIZATION DEPENDS (ALSO) ON THE SAMPLE SIZE!

N of coin tosses	Heads	Tails	Heads/Tails ratio
4	1	3	0,33
10	3	7	0,43
20	8	12	0,67
40	23	17	1,35
100	48	52	0,92
1000	497	503	0,99
2000	998	1002	1

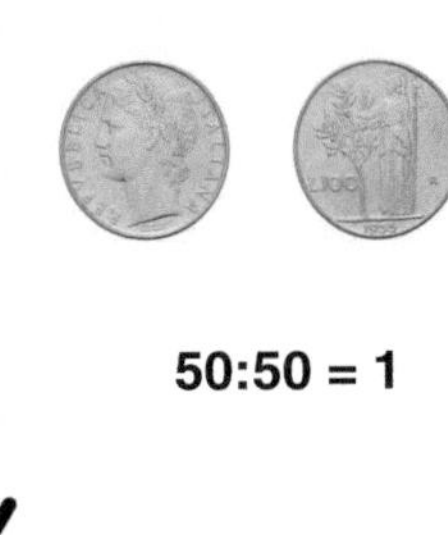

Fig. 15.1 The effectiveness of simple randomization (without restrictions on allocation) in obtaining groups where participants are almost identical in their characteristics depends on the sample size. Larger sample sizes reduce the random variability in group assignment, leading to more balanced groups. Therefore, when designing studies or experiments, researchers often aim for larger sample sizes to enhance the reliability and validity of their findings by minimizing the impact of random chance on group composition

deviate significantly from the expected 50:50 ratio (provided that the coin is not altered and allows for true random allocation) (Fig. 15.1). Thus, in studies conducted in a small number of patients, simple randomization may not adequately balance prognostic factors between the two treatment groups. Block randomization helps ensure that the number of patients enrolled in each group is balanced throughout the study. Alternatively, stratified randomization helps ensure balance for specific prognostic factors, although it may not balance unknown factors.

When evaluating the baseline characteristics of participants assigned to study groups, it's essential to determine whether any observed differences are large enough to be clinically meaningful. If such differences exist, consider how they might have impacted the study results. Which intervention may have been favored or disadvantaged by this imbalance? Additionally, check if the authors made any statistical adjustments to account for these differences.

Sometimes, authors report p-values when presenting baseline characteristics in a table. This practice is incorrect, irrelevant, and potentially misleading. Conceptually, it doesn't make sense to assess the likelihood of differences being due to chance in a randomized study, where participants are assigned to groups randomly. Thus, any differences (or lack thereof) at baseline are expected to be due to chance.

However, this also depends on the level of statistical significance adopted. If the threshold is 0.05, then 5% of statistically significant results could be false positives. Given the high number of variables in the baseline characteristics table, this scenario is quite common. A lack of statistically significant differences may be due to chance. However, it may also be falsely negative, reflecting a small sample size and, consequently, insufficient statistical power to detect a real difference. Statistical power acts like a pair of glasses that helps you detect a difference between two groups, provided that difference truly exists. It is influenced by the sample size: a study with a small sample may lack the power to reveal differences, even if they are present. Insufficient statistical power decreases your visual acuity.

In a randomized controlled trial, statistical power is primarily calculated to identify differences in the study's primary objective, not in the baseline variables compared in the table. Therefore, the statistical power for some baseline characteristics may not be sufficient to detect existing differences. As a result, p-values reported in baseline characteristics tables are often questionable, misleading, and ultimately useless. Instead of relying on p-values, trust your own critical reasoning.

15.2.2 Was the Prognostic Balance Between the Two Groups Maintained Throughout the Study? (Checklist III)

Checklist III: Was the Prognostic Balance Between the Two Groups Maintained Throughout the Study?

Was the prognostic balance between the two groups maintained throughout the study?			
Blinding (performance bias): Are the methods to ensure blinding adequate?)			
Are the methods to ensure blinding adequate?			
Were study personnel aware of group allocation and treatment assignment?	No ☐	Yes ☐	Unclear ☐
Were patients/participants aware of group allocation and treatment assignment?	No ☐	Yes ☐	Unclear ☐
Were the groups treated equally apart from the experimental therapy?	No ☐	Yes ☐	Unclear ☐
Blinding (detection bias): Are the methods to ensure blinding adequate?)			
Are the methods to ensure blinding adequate?			
Were outcome assessors aware of group allocation and treatment assignment?	No ☐	Yes ☐	Unclear ☐
Was the outcome assessed equally in the two groups?	No ☐	Yes ☐	Unclear ☐

15.2.2.1 Notes and Tips

Blinding: Guess what it is? Blinding refers to implementing procedures to prevent someone from being aware of group allocation (and treatment assignment) *after* randomization has occurred. Conversely, allocation concealment takes place *before* randomization (Fig. 15.2).

Selection (allocation) Bias

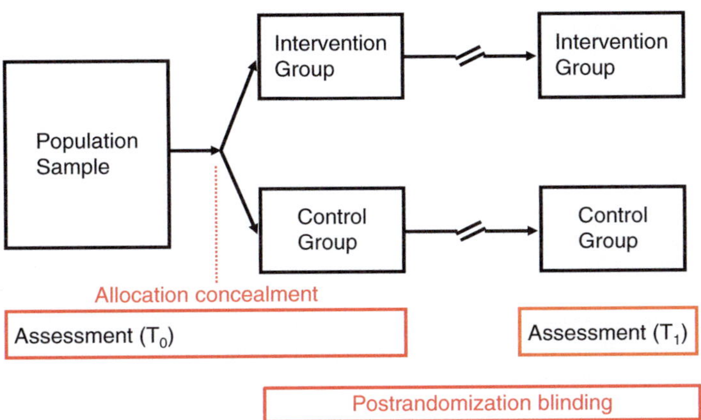

Fig. 15.2 Allocation concealment in randomized controlled trials (RCTs) involves keeping the sequence of participant assignments hidden from those involved in enrolling participants. This is crucial to prevent selection bias, ensuring that allocations are made without prior knowledge or personal preferences influencing the process. Blinding (or masking) in RCTs involves keeping participants, healthcare providers, outcome assessors, and sometimes data analysts unaware of the assigned interventions throughout the study. It aims to prevent performance bias (influencing participant behavior) and detection bias (influencing outcome assessment), thus ensuring that the results are not influenced by knowledge of the treatment assignment. It is important to note that allocation concealment and blinding address biases at different stages of the RCT process: allocation concealment occurs before randomization, while blinding is implemented after randomization has been completed

15.2.3 Were the Two Groups Prognostically Balanced at the End of the Study (Attrition Bias)? (Checklist IV)

Checklist IV: Was the Prognostic Balance Between the Two Groups Maintained Throughout the Study?

Were the two groups prognostically balanced at the end of the study			
Patient loss to follow-up (attrition bias)			
Could the percentage of patients who left the study before its completion and/or were lost to follow-up lead to inaccurate results?	No ☐	Yes ☐	Unclear ☐
Are the reasons for patient loss to follow-up reported?	No ☐	Yes ☐	Unclear ☐
Was the study stopped earlier than expected according to the protocol?	No ☐	Yes ☐	Unclear ☐
Were patients who left the study before its completion and/or were lost to follow-up analyzed in the group to which they had been randomized (intention to treat analysis)?	No ☐	Yes ☐	Unclear ☐

15.2.4 Are There Other Biases? (Checklist V)

Checklist V: Are There Other Biases?

Other biases			
Was the statistical power (and the sample size of the study) calculated?	No ☐	Yes ☐	Unclear ☐
Is there a suspicion of a post hoc selection of the primary outcome (lack of statistical power calculation, no registered protocol)? (*Outcome reporting bias*)	No ☐	Yes ☐	Unclear ☐
In the case of an active comparator, does the study ensure a fair comparison with the experimental treatment, or does it disadvantage it?	No ☐	Yes ☐	Unclear ☐
Could results be biased by economic conflicts of interest (industry-sponsored study, authors employed by the industry, data analysis by the sponsor, etc.)	No ☐	Yes ☐	Unclear ☐

15.2.4.1 Notes and Tips

Statistical power is a pair of glasses. Statistical power can be thought of as a pair of glasses that enables you to discern differences between two groups, assuming those differences truly exist (Fig. 15.3). The effectiveness of these "glasses" relies heavily on various factors, with sample size being one of the most critical. If a study has too few participants, you may fail to detect a genuine difference between groups, even when one is present. Insufficient statistical power reduces your ability to perceive such differences clearly.

In a randomized controlled trial, calculating statistical power is essential to ensure the study can detect differences between groups if they truly exist. This calculation determines the number of participants required for the study to yield meaningful results and should focus on the primary objective, not secondary outcomes.

Fairplay and fair comparisons: it's important to ensure fair play and fair comparisons in the trial. For instance, pay close attention to the dose at which the active comparator is administered, as this can significantly influence the study's findings and their interpretation.

FIND THE DIFFERENCE!

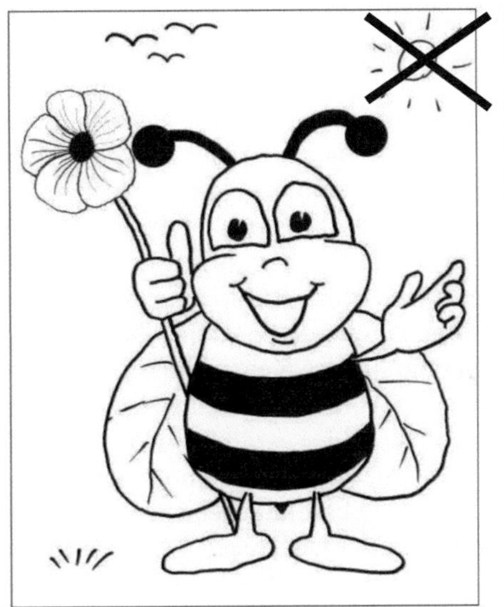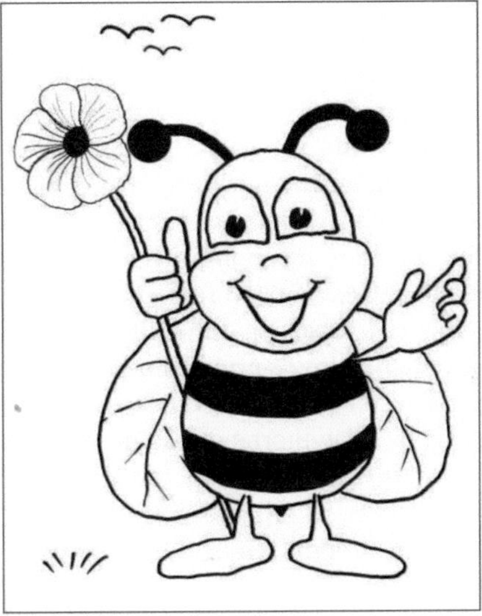

Fig. 15.3 Statistical power is essential for detecting differences between two groups, provided those differences truly exist. The power of a study is largely determined by its sample size. If the sample size is too small, the statistical power may be inadequate to identify a genuine difference, even if one is present. Insufficient statistical power can be likened to having poor visual acuity, which restricts your ability to perceive differences effectively

15.3   What Are the Results? (Checklist VI)

Checklist VI: What Are the Results?

Were comparisons made between groups or within groups?			
Results are reported:			
As absolute values (absolute risk reduction, number needed to treat?	☐		
As risk values (relative risk (risk ratio), relative risk reduction, odds ratio, hazard ratio)?	☐		
Are values reported with precision estimates (confidence intervals)?		No ☐	Yes ☐
How large is the effect size for the treatment?			
Were results statistically significant? Did confidence intervals include the null value?		No ☐	Yes ☐
Was a patient subgroup analysis performed?		No ☐	Yes ☐

15.3.1 Notes and Tips

Compare between, not only within! In any randomized controlled trial, analyses should focus on comparing outcomes between groups rather than only within individual groups. For instance, consider a study comparing the effectiveness of a new migraine drug versus a placebo. Patients with migraines are randomly assigned to receive either the new drug or the placebo. The outcome is measured as the mean number of migraine attacks per month, assessed at baseline and at the trial's conclusion. Patients receiving the new drug report a mean of six migraine attacks per month at baseline and four attacks at the end of the trial, resulting in a mean reduction of two attacks per month within this group. However, this alone does not demonstrate the drug's effectiveness. Changes in migraine frequency within each group could result from various factors, such as natural fluctuations, regression to the mean, the Hawthorne effect, or the placebo effect.

To truly assess the effectiveness of the new drug, a between-group comparison with placebo is necessary. In the placebo group, the baseline frequency is also six attacks per month (indicating successful randomization), decreasing to three attacks per month at the trial's end. This results in an average reduction of three attacks per month in the placebo group. When comparing the average reductions in migraine attacks between the two groups, you find that the placebo group shows a greater reduction (three attacks per month) compared to the new drug group (two attacks per month). This highlights the importance of evaluating outcomes based on the differences between groups, rather than relying solely on differences within each group.

Risk: not always negative—here, the term "risk" carries no negative connotation. It is a neutral term that indicates the probability of an event (outcome) occurring, regardless of whether the outcome is favorable (e.g., drug efficacy) or unfavorable (e.g., mortality).

Measuring imprecision: each study examines only a sample of a population; thus, it is susceptible to sampling error. The results may differ from what would have been observed if the entire population had been studied (sampling error). Confidence intervals, which indicate the range of values likely to include the true value of the underlying population, reflect the level of uncertainty due to this sampling error.

A confidence interval is expressed as a range, with lower and upper bounds indicating its limits. The confidence level, usually a percentage such as 95% or 99%, denotes the probability that the true population parameter lies within the calculated interval. For example, a 95% confidence interval suggests that if the same sample were repeatedly taken, 95% of these intervals would contain the true population parameter.

It's important to remember that a confidence interval provides only an estimation of the true population parameter, and the actual value may lie outside the computed interval. Additionally, the confidence interval does not evaluate the precision of individual measurements or the accuracy of the sampling method.

Statistical significance: statistical significance is typically quantified using a p-value, where "p" stands for probability. p-values indicate the likelihood of obtaining a result equal to or more extreme than the observed result, assuming the null hypothesis is true. The null hypothesis represents the status quo; for instance, it states that there is no difference between treatment and control groups in a randomized controlled trial.

If the p-value is less than a predefined significance level (usually 0.05 or 0.01), the null hypothesis is rejected, leading to the conclusion that there is a statistically significant difference between the groups. A lower p-value suggests stronger evidence against the null hypothesis. For instance, a p-value of 0.001 implies only a 0.1% chance of obtaining a result as extreme or more extreme, assuming the null hypothesis is correct. Such strong evidence may justify rejecting the null hypothesis in favor of the alternative hypothesis (indicating a real difference between groups).

Importantly, in statistical inference, we do not "accept" the null hypothesis; we can only reject it or fail to reject it based on the evidence provided by the data.

The interpretation of p-values can be likened to the force exerted on a scale, where one plate represents the null hypothesis (no difference or no effect) and the other represents the alternative hypothesis (a real difference or effect). A lower p-value tilts the scale toward the alternative hypothesis, indicating stronger support for a genuine difference. Conversely, a higher p-value supports the null hypothesis, suggesting weaker evidence for a difference between groups.

p-values have limitations and should not be used as the sole criterion for determining the significance of a result. They should be interpreted with caution, considering the following:

- The commonly used threshold of 0.05 is merely a convention; more stringent thresholds, such as 0.01, could also be adopted.
- p-values do not provide information about the effect size or the magnitude of the difference between groups; they only reflect a probability.
- p-values do not indicate the clinical relevance of a finding. A small p-value does not necessarily imply clinical significance. Statistical significance does not equate to clinical relevance.
- p-values do not assess the quality of the study or the accuracy of results; they can be influenced by the study methods, risk of confounding, and bias.
- Sample size affects p-values. Larger sample sizes in randomized controlled trials increase the likelihood of detecting statistically significant results, even for small differences between groups. This can lead to lower p-values. Conversely, smaller trials may lack sufficient statistical power to detect smaller differences, resulting in higher p-values.
- Nonsignificant p-values (e.g., >0.05) do not indicate the absence of an effect or difference in the data. Rather, they suggest that the observed data do not provide strong enough evidence to reject the null hypothesis. Such results should be interpreted as "no evidence of a difference" rather than "evidence of no difference."

Null value in confidence intervals: the null value in a confidence interval represents the absence of an effect or difference between two groups. It is commonly used in hypothesis testing to determine if there is a statistically significant difference.

When the null value falls within the calculated confidence interval, it indicates that the difference between the two groups is not statistically significant, and thus the null hypothesis cannot be rejected. Therefore, when interpreting confidence intervals, it is crucial to understand what the null value represents.

For ratios (e.g., risk ratio or odds ratio), the null value is 1. If the confidence interval for the ratio includes the null value of 1, it suggests that there is no significant difference between the groups. If it does not include 1, it indicates a significant difference.

For differences (e.g., mean differences), the null value is 0. If the confidence interval includes 0, it implies no significant difference between the groups. Conversely, if the confidence interval does not include 0, it suggests a significant difference between the groups.

Subgroup results: all that glitters is not gold! Be cautious when interpreting results from subgroup analyses. While a randomized controlled trial (RCT) is typically designed to focus on its primary objective, with sample sizes calculated accordingly, subgroup analyses are often seen as exploratory. Statistically significant findings in subgroup analyses may be spurious (false positives) if adjustments for multiple comparisons have not been made. Even with such adjustments, if the significance level is set at 0.05, statistically significant results can occur by chance in about 5 out of 100 comparisons (or 1 in 20). Therefore, one should be cautious about over-interpreting these results.

Conversely, negative results in subgroup analyses may reflect insufficient statistical power to detect true differences, leading to false negatives. It's essential to recognize that subgroup analyses should not be seen as definitive; rather, any observed differences could be influenced by confounding variables.

While the original study groups are balanced for prognostic factors due to randomization (assuming effective randomization), there is no guarantee that subgroups derived from them will also maintain that balance. Thus, subgroup analyses should be approached with the same caution as observational studies, as they cannot eliminate the possibility of confounding.

15.3.2 Calculation of Results (Table 15.1, Fig. 15.4)

15.3.2.1 Notes and Tips

Relative risk: relative risk (RR) reflects the amount of baseline risk that remains after administering the intervention. It can be compared to the final price after a discount has been applied. A RR of 1 indicates no difference in risk between groups, while a RR less than 1 suggests a reduced risk due to the intervention.

Relative risk reduction: relative risk reduction (RRR) reflects the amount of baseline risk that is removed by the intervention. It can be compared to the discount

Table 15.1 Example of calculation

Event (outcome) rate		Relative risk (risk ratio)	Relative risk reduction (RRR)	Absolute risk reduction (ARR)	Number needed to treat (NNT)
$\dfrac{\text{Control}}{\text{Control event rate}(\text{CER})}$	$\dfrac{\text{Experimental intervention}}{\text{Experimental event rate}(\text{EER})}$	$\dfrac{\text{EER}}{\text{CER}}$	$\dfrac{\text{CER}-\text{EER}}{\text{CER}}$	$\lvert\text{CER}-\text{EER}\rvert$	$\dfrac{1}{\lvert\text{ARR}\rvert}$
9.6%	2.8%	$\dfrac{2.8\%}{9.6\%}=29\%$	$\dfrac{9.6\%-2.8\%}{9.6\%}=71\%$	$\lvert 9.6\%\ -2.8\%\rvert=6.8\%$	$\left\lvert\dfrac{1}{6.8\%}\right\rvert=15$

applied by the vendor. To understand if a certain product is worth purchasing, it's essential to know both the extent of the discount (RRR) and the original price (baseline risk or absolute risk in controls).

Absolute risk reduction: as the name suggests, this is the actual decrease in the risk of an outcome in participants receiving the experimental intervention compared to those in the control group. It is calculated by subtracting the event rate in the control group from that in the experimental group.

Number needed to treat (and number needed to harm): this is the number of patients that need to be treated to observe one positive event (outcome). NNT is always expressed as an integer (if necessary, the number must be rounded to the nearest whole number). Its counterpart is the number needed to harm (NNH): the number of patients that need to be treated to observe one negative event (outcome), such as an adverse effect or death. Under ideal circumstances, *NNT* is equal to 1, indicating that every treated patient experiences a positive outcome.

Consider a randomized controlled trial evaluating the effectiveness of wearing a parachute to prevent death during a jump from a plane. If the survival rate for participants assigned to use a parachute is 100% (experimental event rate), and for those assigned to an "anvil parachute" (as in Wile E. Coyote's cartoons) it is 0% (control event rate), the NNT would be equal to 1. This indicates that treating just one person with the parachute results in one saved life, highlighting the intervention's effectiveness $\left(\dfrac{1}{|\text{ARR}|} = \dfrac{1}{|0\% - 100\%|} = \dfrac{1}{1} = 1 \right)$.

		Relative Risk Reduction RRR	Absolute Risk Reduction ARR	Number Needed to Treat NNT
CER	EER	$\dfrac{\text{CER - EER}}{\text{CER}}$	|CER − EER|	1/|ARR|

Fig. 15.4 Your calculation

15.4 How Can I Apply the Results to My Patients? Assessment of Applicability (External Validity, Generalizability) (Checklist VII)

Checklist VII: How Can I Apply the Results to My Patients?

Patients			
Are the patients and the disease similar enough to those encountered in my clinical practice?	No ☐	Yes ☐	Unclear ☐
Comment:			

Intervention			
Is the intervention applicable to current clinical practice?	No ☐	Yes ☐	Unclear ☐
Comment:			
Outcome(s)			
Have clinically relevant outcomes been considered for the condition in question?	No ☐	Yes ☐	Unclear ☐
Are the likely benefits of the intervention worth the potential harm and costs associated with it?	No ☐	Yes ☐	Unclear ☐

The checklists provided in this chapter have been modified and adapted from materials originally developed by Luca Vignatelli and Maurizio Leone and used in introductory courses on evidence-based practice in Novara and Merano, Italy, with written permission granted for their adaptation.

Further Reading

Guyatt G, Rennie D, Meade MO, Cook DJ, editors. Users' guides to the medical literature: a manual for evidence-based clinical practice. 3rd ed. New York: McGraw-Hill; 2015.
Prasad K. Fundamentals of evidence based medicine. New Delhi: Springer; 2013.

Critical Appraisal of a Therapy Article: Nonrandomized Controlled Study and Uncontrolled Study

16

You can use the following checklists to critically appraise articles reporting the results of nonrandomized controlled and uncontrolled studies (Fig. 16.1). To aid in this process, I've also included a series of notes and tips designed to help you identify methodological flaws in these studies more efficiently. Many of these considerations are similar to those used for appraising randomized controlled trials (see Chap. 15).

Supplementary Information The online version contains supplementary material available at https://doi.org/10.1007/978-3-031-71221-0_16.

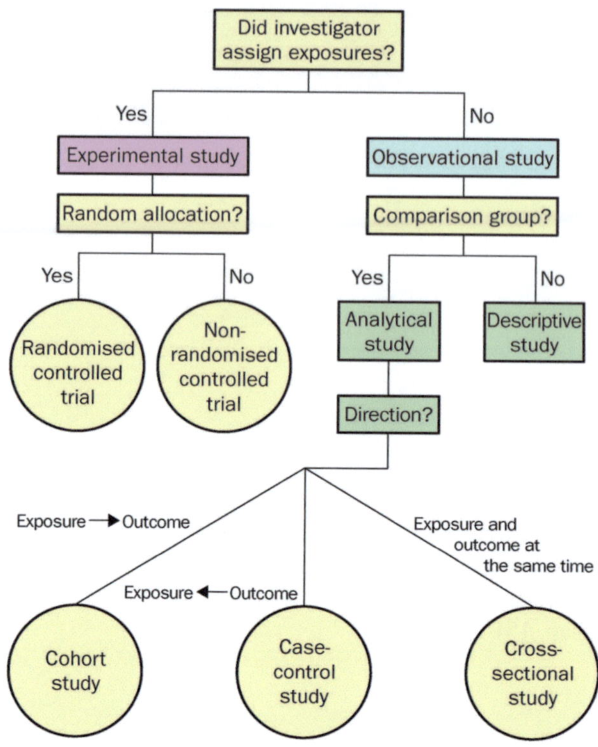

Fig. 16.1 Algorithm for classification of types of clinical research. (Reproduced with permission from: Grimes DA, Schulz KF. An overview of clinical research: the lay of the land. Lancet. 2002;359(9300):57–61)

16.1   Is This Article Relevant to My Clinical Question? (Checklist I)

Checklist I: Is This Article Relevant to My Clinical Question?

Are the patients in the study similar enough to those in my clinical question (clinical characteristics, setting)?	No ☐	Yes ☐	Unclear ☐
Is the intervention evaluated in this study the same as that in my clinical question?	No ☐	Yes ☐	Unclear ☐
Is the intervention evaluated in this study available in my clinical practice?	No ☐	Yes ☐	Unclear ☐
Does this article evaluate the outcome/s I am interested in?	No ☐	Yes ☐	Unclear ☐

16.2 Are the Results Valid? Assessment of Accuracy (Internal Validity, Risk of Bias) (Checklist II)

Checklist II: Are the Results Valid?

Were the patients included consecutively (*selection bias*)?	No ☐	Yes ☐	Unclear ☐
Did the authors adjust results for possible confounders (*confounding*)?	No ☐	Yes ☐	Unclear ☐
Have all factors that could represent confounders been taken into consideration (*confounding*)?	No ☐	Yes ☐	Unclear ☐
For controlled studies: were the participants in the groups treated equally apart from the intervention (no difference in cotreatments) (*performance bias*)?	No ☐	Yes ☐	Unclear ☐
For controlled studies: was the outcome assessed equally in the two groups (*detection bias*)?			
Could the percentage of patients who left the study before its completion and/or were lost to follow-up lead to inaccurate results (*attrition bias*)?	No ☐	Yes ☐	Unclear ☐
Are the reasons for patient loss to follow-up reported (*attrition bias*)?	No ☐	Yes ☐	Unclear ☐
Was the study stopped earlier than expected according to the protocol (*attrition bias*)?	No ☐	Yes ☐	Unclear ☐
Other aspects to consider			
For controlled studies: was the statistical power (and the sample size of the study) calculated?	No ☐	Yes ☐	Unclear ☐
Is there a suspicion of a post hoc selection of the primary outcome (lack of statistical power calculation, no registered protocol) (*outcome reporting bias*)?	No ☐	Yes ☐	Unclear ☐
In the case of an active comparator, does the study ensure a fair comparison with the experimental treatment, or does it disadvantage it?	No ☐	Yes ☐	Unclear ☐
Could results be biased by economic conflicts of interest (industry-sponsored study, authors employed by the industry, data analysis by the sponsor, etc.)	No ☐	Yes ☐	Unclear ☐

16.2.1 Notes and Tips

Consecutive enrollment: excluding patients from a study can introduce selection bias, potentially undermining the validity of the results. This bias could arise when participant selection is nonrandom and influenced by factors related to the study outcome. For example, selectively enrolling patients based on certain characteristics or their likelihood to respond to treatment can lead to confounding by indication (see Chap. 6), impacting the study findings. One effective way to mitigate selection bias is through consecutive enrollment, ensuring that all eligible patients are included.

Confounding: it's important to remember that adjusting for unknown confounding factors is impossible. When interpreting study results, consider other variables, beyond the intervention, that could influence outcomes. Are there additional factors that might have affected prognosis but were not documented or analyzed? A thorough understanding of potential confounders is crucial for accurate interpretation.

Statistical power is a pair of glasses: statistical power can be compared to a pair of glasses that help you discern a difference between two groups, provided such a difference exists. It relies on several factors, with sample size being one of the most important. If a study enrolls too few participants, a genuine difference may go undetected. Insufficient statistical power limits your ability to accurately identify differences. Calculating statistical power in a controlled study is essential to ensure the study can effectively identify differences, particularly for its primary objective.

Fairplay and fair comparisons: ensure that comparisons between groups are conducted fairly, including paying close attention to factors like the dose at which the active comparator was administered. This attention to detail is vital for accurate and meaningful comparisons.

16.3   What Are the Results? (Checklist III)

Checklist III: What Are the Results?

Was there a control group?		No ☐	Yes ☐
For controlled studies: were comparisons made between groups or within groups?			
Results are reported:			
As absolute values (absolute risk reduction, number needed to treat?	☐		
As risk values (relative risk (risk ratio), relative risk reduction, odds ratio, hazard ratio)?	☐		
Are values reported with precision estimates (confidence intervals)?		No ☐	Yes ☐
How large is the effect size for the treatment?			
Were results statistically significant? Did confidence intervals include the null value?		No ☐	Yes ☐
Was a patient subgroup analysis performed?		No ☐	Yes ☐

16.3.1 Notes and Tips

Compared to … nothing! The problems with uncontrolled (before-after) studies: uncontrolled Studies (before-after studies) studies assess the effects of an intervention by comparing outcomes before and after its implementation within the same group. However, this design has significant limitations regarding the ability to draw causal conclusions about the relationship between the exposure (e.g., medication) and outcome (e.g., efficacy). Clinical improvements or positive outcomes could be due to various factors, including the natural course of the disease (e.g., spontaneous remission or improvement), regression to the mean, the Hawthorne effect, and the placebo effect.

As a result, uncontrolled studies inherently provide less reliable results compared to controlled studies. Additionally, the absence of a comparator prevents uncontrolled studies from offering insights into the relative efficacy and safety of a specific intervention.

Compare between, not only within! What truly matters in evaluating outcomes is the difference between groups rather than the difference within each group. Evaluating outcomes effectively requires a clear comparison, as within-group changes can be misleading without a control group to provide context. Refer also to the commentary in the checklist for a critical appraisal of a randomized controlled trial.

Risk: not always negative—here, the term "risk" carries no negative connotation. It is a neutral term that refers to the probability of any event occurring, whether positive or negative. This includes the likelihood of both beneficial outcomes (like efficacy) and adverse events (like mortality).

Measuring imprecision: all studies involve sampling from a population, which introduces the potential for sampling error. This means the results may differ from those that would be obtained by studying the entire population. These intervals provide a range of values within which the true population parameter is likely to fall, reflecting the uncertainty of the sample estimate. A typical confidence level is 95%, meaning that if the study were repeated, 95% of the calculated intervals would contain the true value.

While confidence intervals are useful for estimating population parameters, they do not guarantee precision or accuracy of individual measurements. The true population parameter may fall outside the confidence interval, and the method used to obtain the sample may also introduce bias.

Statistical significance: statistical significance is typically quantified using a p-value, where "p" stands for "probability." p-values indicate the likelihood of obtaining a result equal to or more extreme than the observed result, assuming the null hypothesis is true. The null hypothesis represents the status quo, suggesting no difference between treatment and control groups in a controlled study. If the p-value is less than the chosen significance level (often 0.05 or 0.01), the null hypothesis is rejected. This leads to the conclusion that there is a statistically significant difference between the groups.

A lower p-value indicates stronger evidence against the null hypothesis. For example, a p-value of 0.001 implies only a 0.1% chance of observing a result as extreme as the one observed, assuming the null hypothesis is correct. This strong evidence may justify rejecting the null hypothesis (no real difference between groups) in favor of the alternative hypothesis (real difference between groups).

It is crucial to note that we do not "accept" the null hypothesis; rather, we can either reject it or fail to reject it based on the evidence provided by the data.

The p-value can be likened to the force applied on a balance scale, where one plate represents the null hypothesis (no difference or no effect) and the other represents the alternative hypothesis (real difference or effect). When the p-value is below the significance threshold (e.g., 0.05), it exerts a stronger force on the plate of the alternative hypothesis, pushing it downwards and lending support to the idea of a real difference or effect. The lower the p-value, the stronger the evidence for the alternative hypothesis.

Conversely, if the p-value exceeds the significance threshold, the plate of the null hypothesis holds greater weight. A higher p-value strengthens the null hypothesis, suggesting that observed differences may be due to chance rather than a real effect.

The p-values have limitations and should not be used as the sole criterion for determining the significance of a result. They should be interpreted with caution, considering the following:

- The threshold of 0.05 is commonly used, but it is only a convention. A more extreme threshold could be adopted (e.g., 0.01).
- p-values do not tell anything about the effect size or the strength of the difference between the two groups. It only reflects a probability.
- p-values do not tell anything about the clinical relevance of a finding. For example, a small p-value does not necessarily mean that the result is clinically meaningful. Statistical significance is not synonymous with clinical relevance.
- p-values do not tell anything about the quality of the study or the accuracy of results: they depend on the methods adopted, the risk of confounding, and bias.
- p-values are influenced by sample size. A larger sample size in a controlled study increases the likelihood of finding statistically significant results when there is a real difference between groups. However, with a larger sample, even small differences between groups or effects can become statistically significant, yielding lower p-values. Conversely, controlled studies with small sample sizes may not have enough statistical power (or visual acuity, see above) to detect smaller differences between groups, resulting in higher p-values.
- Nonsignificant p-values (i.e., p-values higher than the statistical threshold, e.g., >0.05) do not necessarily indicate that there is no effect or difference in the data. It means that the observed data do not provide sufficiently strong evidence to reject the null hypothesis. They should be interpreted as "no evidence of a difference" and not be confused with "evidence of no difference."

Null value in confidence intervals: the null value within a confidence interval represents no effect or difference between two groups and is pivotal in hypothesis testing to assess statistical significance. If the null value lies within the calculated confidence interval, it indicates that the observed difference between groups is not statistically significant, and thus, the null hypothesis cannot be rejected. It is crucial to identify the null value when interpreting confidence intervals.

For ratio measures like risk ratio or odds ratio, the null value is typically 1. If the confidence interval includes the null value of 1, it suggests no significant difference between the compared groups. Conversely, if the confidence interval excludes 1, it indicates a significant difference between the groups.

For differences, the null value is 0. If the confidence interval includes 0, there is no significant difference between the groups. Conversely, if the confidence interval does not include the null value of 0, it indicates a significant difference between the groups.

16.3.2 Calculation of Results (Table 16.1, Fig. 16.2)

16.3.2.1 Notes and Tips

Relative risk: relative risk (RR) quantifies the extent to which the baseline risk remains after administering an intervention. It can be likened to the final price obtained after applying a discount to the initial price.

Relative risk reduction: relative risk reduction (RRR) represents the proportion of baseline risk that is mitigated by the intervention, analogous to the discount offered by a vendor. However, determining the value of a product does not solely depend on knowing the extent of the discount (RRR); you also need to be aware of the original price (baseline risk or absolute risk in controls).

Absolute risk reduction: as the name suggests, an absolute reduction in the risk of the event (outcome) in subjects receiving the experimental intervention compared to controls is calculated by subtraction.

Number needed to treat (and number needed to harm): the number needed to treat (NNT) is the number of patients who need to be treated to observe one positive event (outcome). NNT is always an integer and may need to be rounded to the nearest whole number. Conversely, the number needed to harm (NNH) represents the number of patients who need to be treated to observe one negative event (outcome), such as adverse effects or death. Ideally, an *NNT* of 1 indicates that every patient treated experiences a positive outcome. For more information, refer to Chap. 15.

Table 16.1 Example of calculation

Event (outcome) rate		Relative risk (risk ratio)	Relative risk reduction (RRR)	Absolute risk reduction (ARR)	Number needed to treat (NNT)
$\dfrac{\text{Control}}{\text{Control event rate}(\text{CER})}$	$\dfrac{\text{Experimental intervention}}{\text{Experimental event rate}(\text{EER})}$	$\dfrac{\text{EER}}{\text{CER}}$	$\dfrac{\text{CER}-\text{EER}}{\text{CER}}$	$\lvert\text{CER}-\text{EER}\rvert$	$\dfrac{1}{\lvert\text{ARR}\rvert}$
9.6%	2.8%	$\dfrac{2.8\%}{9.6\%}=29\%$	$\dfrac{9.6\%-2.8\%}{9.6\%}=71\%$	$\lvert 9.6\%\ -2.8\%\rvert=6.8\%$	$\left\lvert\dfrac{1}{6.8\%}\right\rvert=15$

		Relative Risk Reduction	Absolute Risk Reduction	Number Needed to Treat
		RRR	ARR	NNT
CER	EER	$\dfrac{CER - EER}{CER}$	|CER – EER|	1/|ARR|

Fig. 16.2 Your calculation

16.4 How Can I Apply the Results to My Patients? Assessment of Applicability (External Validity, Generalizability) (Checklist IV)

Checklist IV: How Can I Apply the Results to My Patients?

Patients			
Are the patients and the disease similar enough to those encountered in my clinical practice?	No ☐	Yes ☐	Unclear ☐
Comment:			

Intervention			
Is the intervention applicable to current clinical practice?	No ☐	Yes ☐	Unclear ☐
Comment:			

Outcome(s)			
Have clinically relevant outcomes been considered for the condition in question?	No ☐	Yes ☐	Unclear ☐
Are the likely benefits of the intervention worth the potential harm and costs associated with it?	No ☐	Yes ☐	Unclear ☐

The checklists included in this chapter have been modified and adapted from materials originally developed by Luca Vignatelli and Maurizio Leone. These resources were used in introductory courses on evidence-based practice in Novara and Merano, Italy, with written permission granted for their adaptation.

Further Reading

Guyatt G, Rennie D, Meade MO, Cook DJ, editors. Users' guides to the medical literature: a manual for evidence-based clinical practice. 3rd ed. New York: McGraw-Hill; 2015.
Prasad K. Fundamentals of evidence based medicine. New Delhi: Springer; 2013.

You can use the following checklists to critically appraise an article on diagnosis. To further facilitate this task, I have included a series of notes and tips to identify methodological flaws in diagnostic articles more efficiently and effectively. Details on the diagnostic process and parameters (such as sensitivity, specificity, positive and negative predictive values, and positive and negative likelihood ratios) are discussed in Chap. 10, while systematic errors (biases) that can occur in diagnostic studies are covered in Chap. 11.

17.1   Is This Article Relevant to My Clinical Question? (Checklist I)

Checklist I: Is This Article Relevant to My Clinical Question?

Are the patients in the study similar enough to those of my clinical question (clinical characteristics, setting)?	No ☐	Yes ☐	Unclear ☐
Is the diagnostic test under investigation relevant to my clinical question?	No ☐	Yes ☐	Unclear ☐
Is the diagnostic test available in my clinical practice?	No ☐	Yes ☐	Unclear ☐
Does this article aim to establish the diagnostic ability of this test?	No ☐	Yes ☐	Unclear ☐

Supplementary Information The online version contains supplementary material available at https://doi.org/10.1007/978-3-031-71221-0_17.

17.2 Are the Results Valid? Assessment of Accuracy (Internal Validity, Risk of Bias) (Checklist II)

Checklist II: Are the Results Valid?

Patient selection			
Patient selection is based on:			
Results of reference standard bias (*referral bias*)	☐		
Case-control design (*spectrum bias*)	☐		
Consecutive series	☐		
Not described/unclear	☐		
Were patients with unclear or indeterminate test results (including borderline results or findings that are technically difficult to evaluate) excluded (*spectrum bias*)?	No ☐	Yes ☐	Unclear ☐
Index test			
Were the test results interpreted without knowledge of the reference standard results (*review bias*)?	No ☐	Yes ☐	Unclear ☐
Reference standard			
Is the reference standard appropriate?	No ☐	Yes ☐	Unclear ☐
Were the results of the reference standard interpreted without knowledge of the results of the index test?	No ☐	Yes ☐	Unclear ☐
Did only some patients receive the reference standard test, with the other patients not receiving any reference standard test (*partial verification bias*)?	No ☐	Yes ☐	Unclear ☐
Were two different reference standard tests used, depending on whether the index test was positive or negative (*differential verification bias*)?	No ☐	Yes ☐	Unclear ☐
Were the results of the index test incorporated into the reference standard test (*incorporation bias*)?	No ☐	Yes ☐	Unclear ☐
Study flow			
Is the interval between the index test and the reference standard appropriate (is there a risk that the condition has changed in the meantime)?	No ☐	Yes ☐	Unclear ☐
Were all patients included in the analysis?	No ☐	Yes ☐	Unclear ☐

17.3 What Are the Results? (Checklist III)

Checklist III: What Are the Results?

Have diagnostic accuracy parameters been reported?	No ☐	Yes ☐
Are diagnostic parameters reported with precision estimates (confidence intervals)?	No ☐	Yes ☐
Was a patient subgroup analysis performed?	No ☐	Yes ☐

17.3.1 Notes and Tips

Measuring imprecision: each study examines only a sample of a population and is therefore subject to sampling error. The results obtained from the sample may differ from what would have been observed if the study had been conducted on the entire population from which the sample was drawn (sampling error). Confidence intervals, which indicate the range of values likely to include the true value of the underlying population, reflect the degree of uncertainty due to sampling error.

17.3.2 Calculation of Diagnostic Parameters (Table 17.1)

17.3.3 Notes and Tips

Pretest probability: pretest probability is the likelihood that an individual has a disease before any diagnostic test is performed. Suppose it is known that about 7 out of 100 individuals in a certain population have disease X. If we randomly select an individual from this population (to avoid selection bias) and conduct a diagnostic test to determine if they have disease X, the pretest probability that they have the disease would be 7% or 0.07.

Pretest odds: pretest odds are a measure of the likelihood of having a disease before a diagnostic test is performed. It is calculated by dividing the pretest probability of having the disease by the probability of not having the disease. For example, suppose the pretest probability of having a certain disease is 0.2 or 20%, then the pretest odds of having the disease would be $0.2/(1 - 0.2) = 0.25$. The reason we use pretest odds instead of pretest probability is that odds can be transformed into a

Table 17.1   Calculation of diagnostic parameters

		Condition of interest		Total
Results of the diagnostic test		Presente	Assente	
	Positive	a	b	$a + b$
	Negative	c	d	$c + d$
	Total	$a + c$	$b + d$	$a + b + c + d$

Sensitivity = $a/(a + c)$ =
Specificity = $d/(b + d)$ =
Positive likelihood ratio (likelihood ratio for a positive result) = LR+ = sens/(1 − spec) =
Negative likelihood ratio (likelihood ratio for a positive result) = LR- = (1 − sens)/spec =
Positive predictive value = $a/(a + b)$ =
Negative predictive value = $d/(c + d)$ =
Pretest probability (prevalence of the condition) = $(a + c)/(a + b + c + d)$ =
Pretest odd = prevalence/(1 − prevalence) =
Posttest odd = pretest odd × likelihood ratio =
Posttest probability = posttest odd/(posttest odd + 1) =

linear scale while probabilities cannot. This transformation allows us to calculate posttest probability using pretest odds and likelihood ratios.

A likelihood ratio measures how much the odds of a disease increase or decrease given a positive or negative test result. For instance, a positive likelihood ratio (given a positive result) of 13 means that the odds of having the disease increased by a factor of 13 if the test result was positive. Posttest odds are then converted to posttest probabilities to make the results of diagnostic tests more easily interpretable.

Posttest odds: posttest odds are a measure of the likelihood of a disease given a positive or negative test result. They are calculated by dividing the probability of having the disease after the test by the probability of not having the disease after the test.

Posttest probability: posttest probability refers to the probability that an individual who tests positive on a diagnostic test actually has the disease. Unlike posttest odds, which are ratios, posttest probabilities directly represent the likelihood of having the disease after the test has been performed. Posttest odds are typically converted to posttest probabilities to facilitate the interpretation of diagnostic test results. Aside from the process of converting pretest probability to pretest odds, using the likelihood ratio to calculate posttest odds, and then converting back to probability, an alternative method is the use of the Fagan nomogram (Fig. 17.1).

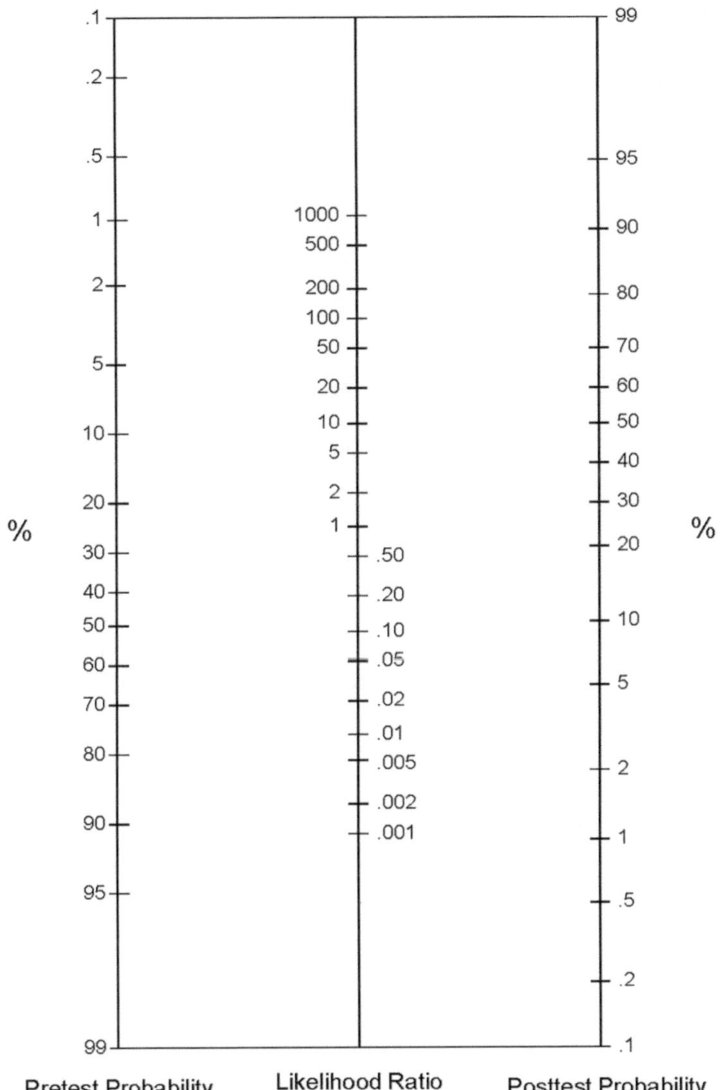

Fig. 17.1 A Fagan nomogram is a graphical tool used in medicine to estimate posttest probabilities based on diagnostic test results. It incorporates the pretest probability of a condition and the test's sensitivity and specificity. To use the Fagan nomogram, one draws a line from the estimated pretest probability (on the left axis) through the likelihood ratio (LR) corresponding to the observed test result (in the center). The point where this line intersects the right axis indicates the posttest probability. The Fagan nomogram is particularly valuable for quickly interpreting test results without extensive calculations. This visual aid helps in making informed decisions about further diagnostic or therapeutic actions, incorporating test characteristics directly into the interpretation process. The Fagan nomogram was originally described by Thomas B. Fagan in his article titled *Nomogram for Bayes's Theorem*, published in 1975 in The New England Journal of Medicine. This article introduced this graphical tool as a method to apply Bayes' theorem in medical decision-making, particularly for interpreting diagnostic test results and estimating posttest probabilities. (Source: Wikipedia Commons (Author: Eric Youngstrom). Figure licensed under the Creative Commons Attribution-Share Alike 4.0 International license)

17.4 How Can I Apply the Results to My Patient? Assessment of Applicability (External Validity, Generalizability) (Checklist IV)

Checklist IV: How Can I Apply the Results to My Patient?

Are the patients in the study similar enough to those in my clinical practice (patient selection, clinical characteristics, setting)?	No ☐	Yes ☐	Unclear ☐
Is the diagnostic test available and cost-effective in my clinical practice?	No ☐	Yes ☐	Unclear ☐
Is the level of acceptance of the test higher than or equal to that of other diagnostic tests?	No ☐	Yes ☐	Unclear ☐
Will the test result (resulting posttest probabilities) change my treatment choice?	No ☐	Yes ☐	Unclear ☐
Will patients benefit from the results of this test (i.e., is there an effective therapy for the disease or condition I am trying to diagnose)?	No ☐	Yes ☐	Unclear ☐

The checklists included in this chapter have been modified and adapted from materials originally developed by Luca Vignatelli and Maurizio Leone. These resources were used in introductory courses on evidence-based practice in Novara and Merano, Italy, with written permission granted for their adaptation.

Further Reading

Guyatt G, Rennie D, Meade MO, Cook DJ, editors. Users' guides to the medical literature: a manual for evidence-based clinical practice. 3rd ed. New York: McGraw-Hill; 2015.
Prasad K. Fundamentals of evidence based medicine. New Delhi: Springer; 2013.

Part III

Epilogue

Beware of Masters (Yes, Even of Charcot)! The Importance of Distrusting Everything and Everyone

18

Remember that your teachers are as full of bullshit as your parents.

—*David Sackett (1934–2015)*

It is crucial to approach' medicine with a healthy dose of skepticism and to question tradition and authorities. This chapter highlights the risks of blindly trusting medical authorities and emphasizes the importance of continuously asking questions, seeking answers, and testing the validity of expert opinions. This mindset fosters curiosity and intellectual freedom.

Unlike other chapters, this one does not begin with a quote by Charcot, the master. The reason is straightforward: no teacher would ever accept the notion that they could be wrong—much less entertain the horrifying idea of being... full of bullshit! With due respect to my own teachers and parents, I will discuss the role of tradition in medicine and the limitations and risks of an overly trusting approach toward medical authorities, urging you to maintain a healthy skepticism about everything, including Charcot himself.

Herein, I propose a less than reverent interpretation of the famous painting *La Leçon Clinique à la Salpêtrière* (A Clinical Lesson at the Salpêtrière) by André Brouillet (1857–1914) (Fig. 18.1). In this work, Charcot is depicted delivering a clinical lecture to a large audience. A hysterical patient, Marie Wittman (known as "Blanche" (1859–1912)), leans unconsciously against Charcot's pupil, Joseph Babiński (1857–1932), while the spectators gaze attentively at Charcot. The issue, however, is that none of the physicians in attendance are truly focused on her; they are mesmerized by Charcot's authority—his voice, his expression, and his gestures. Nobody seems to really pay attention to the patient. Everyone is looking, but no one is truly seeing. By fixating on the master's authority, they miss the reality before them.

F. Brigo, *Charcot's Lesson*, Neurocultural Health and Wellbeing, https://doi.org/10.1007/978-3-031-71221-0_18

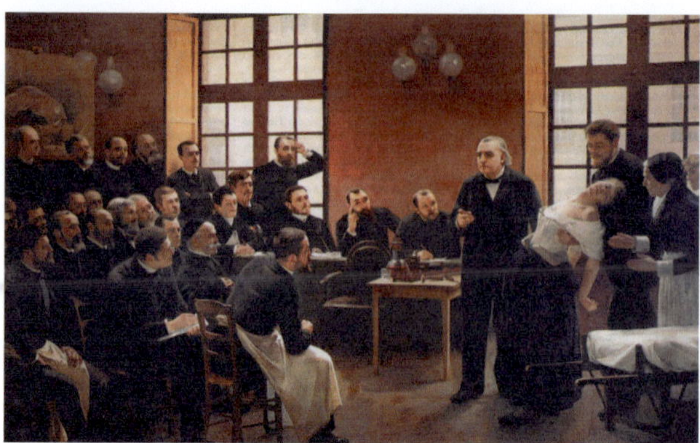

Fig. 18.1 André Brouillet's painting "Une leçon clinique à la Salpêtrière" portrays a significant scene from the clinical lectures conducted by Jean-Martin Charcot at the Salpêtrière Hospital in Paris during the late nineteenth century. The painting depicts Charcot leading a clinical demonstration, surrounded by medical students and doctors in a lecture hall

Admittedly, this interpretation does not capture the painter's true intent, which was likely to pay sincere homage to the great French neurologist and his pupils. However, it serves as an appropriate entry point for discussing the theme of authority and authoritativeness in medicine.

For centuries, from antiquity through the Middle Ages and beyond, medicine was rooted in accumulated knowledge centered on the teachings of key figures whose influence shaped clinical practice. This created a mental straitjacket, stifling creativity and experimentation, and forcing physicians to view health, disease, patients, and disorders through the narrow lens of medical tradition. The authoritative—often authoritarian—opinions of Galen and his followers dominated the interpretation of reality, impeding advances in anatomy and physiology. It is surprising to consider how limited and biased physicians' perspectives were, even during autopsies. It is hard to imagine that no one dared to question what a lecturer stated, quoting Galen and other historical authorities. Much like in Andersen's folktale, we might wish someone would boldly declare the truth: "The emperor is wearing no clothes! Galen is wrong!"

It seems history is not to blame; we cannot evaluate the past through present paradigms. However, it is undeniable that the cultural systems of antiquity and the Middle Ages were relatively closed, self-referential, and rigid due to religious, political, social, and anthropological motivations. While these forces were present, they appear less pronounced than in later historical periods. Ultimately, it took the restless and curious gaze of Renaissance thinkers to penetrate the rigid theoretical armor of medieval medicine, allowing them to see reality anew. But why did this transformation take so long? Beyond the historical factors, I believe there is a deeper issue rooted in human psychology: relying on others is often reassuring and comfortable.

As children, we tend to believe our parents are always right. As teenagers, we grow, rebel, and seek independence, believing that severing ties with past authority figures allows us to master ourselves and make independent judgments. Yet, as social beings, we have an inherent tendency to trust those we respect. In my early days at work, faced with clinical procedures I questioned, I once asked a colleague why we followed certain practices. The response echoed a sentiment that has persisted through centuries of medicine: "He (the boss) said so. Stop questioning and just do it! He knows what needs to be done; you can trust his experience!"

We often rely on authority figures, as following their lead earns us approval and spares us the effort of considering alternatives. So why should we challenge authority? The answer is simple: everyone, even experts, makes mistakes and can be mistaken—often without realizing it. Knowledge derived from clinical experience may be limited, outdated, or unsupported by evidence. Research studies can also be biased, intentionally or unintentionally. False theories and cognitive biases distort reality, influenced by personal beliefs, financial interests, or political agendas. Thus, it is no surprise that expert opinion occupies the lowest tier of the evidence-based medicine pyramid. While expert opinion is unquestionably valuable, its worth is limited, especially when stronger evidence is available. All expert statements must be scrutinized through the lens of evidence, reinforcing the motto of the Royal Society: *Nullius in verba* (take nobody's word for it).

Continuously asking questions, seeking answers, and verifying the robustness and validity of expert opinions cultivates a spirit of curiosity and preserves intellectual freedom. In medicine, no authority should be obeyed without question. When in the presence of authority, remember to remove your hat—but please, don't take off your head.

Notwithstanding the details I have already provided, I am far from having exhausted the subject, and I dare to hope that you will not regret the time yet remaining to be dedicated to its study.

—Jean-Martin Charcot, *Leçons sur les Maladies du Système Nerveux faites a la Salpêtrière*. Volume 1, Lecture II. Paris, 1877

Index

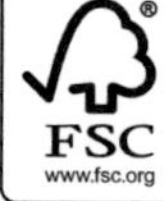